# The Healthy Low GI Low Carb Diet

**DR CHARLES CLARK
& MAUREEN CLARK**

**Vermilion**
LONDON

5 7 9 10 8 6 4

Copyright © Dr Charles Clark and Maureen Clark 2005

First published in the United Kingdom in 2005 by Vermilion,
an imprint of Ebury Publishing,
Random House UK Ltd.
Random House
20 Vauxhall Bridge Road
London SW1V 2SA

Random House Australia (Pty) Limited
20 Alfred Street, Milsons Point, Sydney,
New South Wales 2061, Australia

Random House New Zealand Limited
18 Poland Road, Glenfield,
Auckland 10, New Zealand

Random House (Pty) Limited
Endulini, 5A Jubilee Road, Parktown 2193, South Africa

Random House UK Limited Reg. No. 954009
www.randomhouse.co.uk
Papers used by Vermilion are natural, recyclable products made from
wood grown in sustainable forests.

A CIP catalogue record is available for this book from the British Library.

ISBN: 0091902541

Designed by Two Associates

Printed and bound in Great Britain by
Bookmarque Limited, Croydon, Surrey

The advice offered in this book is not intended to be a substitute for the advice
and counsel of your personal physician. Always consult a medical practitioner
before embarking on a diet, or a course of exercise. Neither the authors nor the
publisher can be held responsible for any loss or claim arising out of the use,
or misuse, of the suggestions made, or the failure to take medical advice.

# Contents

# Acknowledgements

Once again we acknowledge the essential role of our children, David and Heather, in the final format of our books. Children provide probably the most severe test for any author on food matters. They can be devastatingly critical, and in this regard our children are world champions. However, the criticism is almost always innocently frank and honest and therefore usually highly relevant. To encourage children to actually *enjoy* healthy foods from the outset is our major challenge because if we can achieve this then many of the diseases which are a direct result of poor diet will simply not occur.

The secret of effective medicine is prevention rather than cure and this can only be achieved by the encouragement of a healthy lifestyle from the earliest possible moment.

# Introduction

There is currently a plethora of low-carb diets on the market –
including a very successful diet by the authors of this book – so
how does this one differ? The plain fact is that low-carb diets,
although all based on the simple principle of reducing carbohydrates rather than calories, are actually different from each
other. However, the aim of this book is to simplify the process of
understanding the principle of low-carb dieting and to explain a
diet that is complementary to our current books, which allows
everyone to enjoy a low-carb lifestyle. It explains the close
association between a healthy low-carb diet (which restricts
*refined* carbohydrates but not *unrefined* carbohydrates) and a
low glycaemic index (or low-GI) diet, in so doing incorporating
all the diverse groups of dieters who were previously excluded
from the typical low-carb regime, primarily vegetarians and
those who enjoy pasta, rice, grains and fruit. All of these
delicious foods *are* included in this low-carb diet.

And the most important principle is to keep it simple – because
a healthy diet is simple! To be successful, a diet must be:

- Easy to follow
- Tasty and enjoyable
- Satisfying – which means you are not hungry
- Healthy – including all of the essential nutrition you
  require
- Effective in losing excess weight – but not causing loss
  of body protein (which occurs in excessive low-calorie
  diets)

The healthy low-GI/low-carb diet is low in refined carbohydrates but includes virtually all other foods – and we mean *all* other foods: poultry, fish, shellfish, pasta, rice, fruit, vegetables, wholegrains, dairy products and eggs. (Red meat, however, is the exception, for reasons explained below.) It is based on medically proven principles and has been shown to be very effective, not only in achieving easy and sustainable weight loss, but also in the prevention of diabetes, the lowering of blood lipids and therefore the prevention of heart disease.

Some diets are based on the principle of reducing *all* carbohydrates to very low levels, usually less than 20 grams per day, at least in the initial stages. Lowering carbohydrate intake will lower levels of the hormone insulin, which effectively is the controlling mechanism for building fat from calories. So an inevitable consequence is that lowering carbohydrate levels to this degree will maximise the weight-loss effect of the diet.

But unfortunately there are many natural *unrefined* carbohydrates, such as those present in fruit and vegetables, which are also combined with the vitamins and minerals we need for health. These vitamins and minerals are absolutely essential for our continued health and well-being, and without them we will undoubtedly become malnourished and unwell. Diets which severely restrict all carbohydrates (including those in vegetables) usually advise multivitamin supplements to make up the shortfall in essential nutrients, and this is certainly a method of preventing ill-health from malnutrition as a direct result of the diet.

We do not advocate this approach. Firstly, there is no guarantee in vitamin and mineral supplements that you will obtain all of the nutrients essential for health, and secondly it is not known whether the vitamins and minerals in supplements are as effective as those present in their natural environment: fruit and vegetables. There is, however, no scientific doubt that vitamins and minerals present in fresh fruit and vegetables are not only in their highest concentration, but also in their most effective chemical format as essential components of our diet. So fresh fruit and vegetables are an integral component of this healthy diet.

Why should you choose this low-GI/low-carbohydrate diet instead of the more conventional low-calorie diet? Simply because it works – unlike the multitude of low-calorie diets available – *and it is healthy*. The health aspects will be described in detail in Chapters 5 and 6. The principles are easy to follow and require virtually no will-power.

This low-GI/low-carb diet has been specifically designed to include only foods that are universally accepted to be healthy, such as vegetables, fruit, fish, poultry and essential fatty acids. We have deliberately omitted red meat and restricted dairy products and eggs to reduce the levels of saturated fats in the diet to minimal proportions. This does not imply that these foods are *unhealthy*, merely that we have deliberately *only* included foods which have no contentious elements whatsoever, to prove that a low-carb diet need not include unacceptable levels of saturated fats, and certainly need not exclude fruit and vegetables. In other words, it is to prove – once and for all – that a low-carb diet is *not* unhealthy, and does not exclude fruit and vegetables. And also to prove that a low-carb diet can exclude meat and also be low in saturated fats.

Whilst this book can be used in isolation to provide a healthy low-carb diet, it is intended to complement *The New High Protein Diet* series we have published to date. It is impossible to summarise in a single volume the wealth of knowledge and potential variations in low-carb diets that would be suitable for everyone. We each have individual tastes and pressures upon us which make up the myriad potential lifestyles which any diet must incorporate to be accepted universally. But in a comple-mentary series of books one can encompass the many different lifestyles, varying from those who enjoy meat to those who are vegetarian, from those enjoying traditional home-cooking to the exotic tastes of a wide range of Asian foods – even those to whom a fast-food existence is the norm, either by choice or necessity. Previous books in this series include *The New High Protein Diet*, *The New High Protein Diet Cookbook* and *The New High Protein Healthy Fast Food Diet* (published by Vermilion). We have referred to recipes and low-carb alternatives that are described in the complementary books in the series to provide the widest possible variety of options available in your diet and to avoid any unnecessary repetition.

We know from the many communications we receive that there are numerous low-carb devotees throughout the world who have followed our system and we have attempted to make each new book in the series complementary to those already published to provide the most extensive range of low-GI/low-carb dietary options available.

The recipes in *The Healthy Low GI Low Carb Diet* are completely different as meat has been excluded, whilst fruit, grains, pasta, rice, pulses and dairy products are included.

**The essential difference, of course, is that the inclusion of these foods containing higher proportions of carbohydrates means that the individual must count the carbohydrates in each individual meal.**

There is a varied range of recipes including rice or pasta with an extensive use of vegetables as both main meals or side dishes, so this diet has the unique advantage of being the first low-GI/low-carb diet that is equally suitable for vegetarians. The only proviso we would emphasise is that vegetarians who do not include eggs in their diet must take Vitamin $B^{12}$ supplements, as this vitamin is not present in foods of plant origin and deficiency will lead to pernicious anaemia.

The advantages in so doing are that every healthy food may now be included in a low-GI/low-carb diet; only unhealthy foods are excluded.

How does the advice given in this book differ from that in other books in the series? Simply because it includes all of the foods which have previously been excluded from a low-carb diet: pasta, rice, bread, pulses, wholegrains and fruit – all in moderation – by taking into account their GI values.

In other words, this form of low-carb diet is the most versatile yet devised. It can be adapted to literally every lifestyle. In previous books we have shown how to follow the diet with meat-based products (*The New High Protein Diet*, *The New High Protein Diet Cookbook*) or even using healthy fast foods which are readily available (*The Healthy Fast Food Diet*). Now it has been adapted to include all foods – with the specific exclusion of red meat to prove this is certainly not prerequisite for a healthy low-carb diet.

Another essential difference between this book and most other low-carb texts is the inclusion of delicious puddings. We have not used carbohydrate substitutes in the recipes; if sugar is necessary it has been included in its pure form in low concentration. So by avoiding artificial sweeteners, there is no possibility of potential adverse effects, about which there has been speculation from time to time.

For the first time, everyone can now enjoy the health benefits and dietary advantages of the low-GI/low-carb lifestyle – and the health benefits are much more extensive than merely loss of weight (desirable as that may be), as will be described later in the book.

# Chapter 1 Why diet?

Why do we diet? Surely the answer is obvious: we diet to be slim and therefore more attractive, either to ourselves or to others. Because, undeniably, to be the 'proud' possessor of excess body fat is considered a grave offence against our cosmetic sensitivities and, more importantly, to those into whose unfortunate gaze we allow our offensive appearance to fall.

In fact, we should all diet to be *healthy*. The advantage of this diet is that you will slim and be healthy at the same time. And it will be both easy and require virtually no will-power as you will be enjoying healthy foods in 'normal' quantities. On the health aspect, this is not yet another platitude without foundation; on the contrary, there is incontrovertible objective medical evidence to substantiate the claim, detailed in Chapter 5. In brief, you will reduce the risks of heart disease, diabetes, arthritis and obesity by using this diet. Major claims – but ones which can be supported.

When we shed the excess kilos (and only the *excess* kilos, as some body fat is normal) we should feel healthier with more energy and increased immunity to infection. And that is really the basis for dieting, because most low-calorie diets *do not* make you feel healthier, but rather the contrary. Because you are consuming far fewer calories than you need, you are constantly weak with hunger. Much worse than that scenario is the fact that you are not consuming enough of the nutrients that you require from food, such as vitamins, minerals, proteins and essential fats. And to make the situation even worse from a health perspective, when the human body enters 'starvation' mode (which is essentially all that a low-calorie diet is) your body naturally starts to break down body proteins, which is definitely unhealthy.

In other words, a diet which is effective in weight loss should also be effective in promoting health, and any diet in which you lose weight in the process of becoming unhealthy is nothing short of absurd.

Dieting has become an integral part of life for many individuals in Western society. The urge to be slim, preferably whilst still enjoying the 'pleasures' of life, is, in many ways, the typical Western lifestyle. And for most people the diet is not successful, either because it is impossible to follow, or because the individual cannot adhere to an impossible regime.

This was certainly the usual course of events until recently. Or, more precisely, until the era of the *low-carbohydrate diet*. Unlike its rival, the low-fat or low-calorie diet, the dieter does not have to restrict calories on this diet and therefore is never hungry. Whilst certainly restricting some of the more 'delicious' gastronomic pleasures in life – cakes, biscuits and even (heaven forbid) chips – it allows large quantities of relatively unrestricted foods that also have the advantage of being very enjoyable.

Low-carb diets are assumed to be a relatively new phenomenon, but the concept has been promoted for almost a century. It is only recently that the diet has gained in popularity, and for very good reason, as it is a conceptual method of dieting which has considerable medical evidential basis for success.

Unfortunately there are many different low-carb diets available, many of which concentrate entirely on the weight-loss aspect and ignore the necessity to provide all of the essential nutrients for health. That is the prime *raison d'être* for this diet; it encapsulates all of the knowledge we have acquired to provide a successful weight-loss programme that also incorporates all of the essential nutrients for health.

A nutritionally balanced diet is absolutely essential for health for various good reasons, not just weight, which is merely one (although perhaps the most obvious) aspect of poor diet. Our bodies cope with immense insults from poor lifestyle over many years, until eventually they collapse with multisystem failure as the heart, lungs, joints and nervous system are unable to cope with continued demands. Most of these problems can be prevented to a large extent by a healthy lifestyle. In most cases, heart disease, diabetes, arthritis and hypertension can be avoided by changes in the way we live. The problem is that most people leave these changes too late. The secret is to allow your lifestyle to *prevent* disease occurring, not to try to use diet to *treat* the disease, as by this stage there is a variable amount of permanent damage. And enjoying a healthy diet does not mean living a frugal, monkish existence. On the contrary, you can enjoy delicious foods in adequate quantities, and the healthy constituents in the food will be actually improving your health and vitality, rather than gradually eroding your health – which is the consequence of many of the most popular high-carbohydrate foods, the basis of the 'Western' diet.

In a 'modern' society, we are constantly bombarded with increased choice in the food market. In reality, whilst the *variety* of foods has increased, the *choice* of healthy foods is probably more restricted than at any time in our history. So much food has been processed in ways which are difficult to detect that we are simply not sure what we are *actually* consuming, as opposed to what we *assume* we are consuming. The additives and preservatives in pre-packaged foods and processed foods are obvious, as they are detailed on the packaging. Less obvious is the fact that many packaged and processed foods contain very little of the essential nutrition which we require to maintain health. In reality, most pre-packaged 'fast' foods comprise mainly refined carbohydrates and fats, which have the triple dubious advantages of being filling, very cheap to produce (if not to purchase) and, by inducing surges of insulin in the body, also highly addictive.

This book will demonstrate how you can identify and incorporate all of the healthy foods which are readily available, to ensure your diet is both successful (in terms of weight loss) and healthy.

# Chapter 2

## Insulin – the key to health and successful weight loss

There has been considerable press on the role of insulin in low-carb diets but our clinical experience is that many patients have found some of the explanations difficult to understand or simply inaccurate. This is unfortunate, as an understanding of the role of insulin is central to both successful weight loss and returning your body to health. We have tried to simplify the explanation of the role of insulin in this chapter. And the role of insulin is certainly not difficult to understand.

Insulin is a hormone produced by an organ called the pancreas. It has profound effects on every cell in the body. Production of insulin is stimulated by carbohydrates in our diet, and to a much lesser degree by protein. It is not stimulated by fats in the diet.

So far, so good. But what is the role of insulin and why is it so bad?

The first point to emphasise is that insulin *per se* is not bad; in fact, a certain amount of insulin is absolutely essential for health. The problem is that our modern diet stimulates the production of far too much.

Let us now consider the adverse effects of producing too much insulin.

Firstly, and most relevant to dieting, insulin causes excess calories to be stored as fat. Even worse, it actually prevents the breakdown of fat cells. So not only does insulin stimulate the production of fat (which you are trying to lose) but it also prevents the use of your stored fat as energy. Now you can understand why you must reduce insulin production if your diet is to be successful.

But the adverse effects on health of excess insulin are much worse than merely the storage of excess fat. They include:

- Excess production of cholesterol by the liver, causing raised cholesterol levels and increasing the risk of heart disease
- Stimulating the kidneys to retain excess water and salt, which can lead to raised blood pressure
- Increasing the muscular component of the walls of arteries, which further contributes to high blood pressure
- Increasing the levels of fats in the blood called 'triglycerides', which are a very significant indicator of heart disease

It is instantly apparent that excess insulin is very undesirable indeed.

But just when you think the situation cannot get worse, it does! As we make more and more insulin in response to more and more carbohydrates in our diet, the cells of the body become less responsive to these excessive amounts of hormone. The cells become resistant to insulin and the condition of *insulin resistance* develops. And as the cells become more resistant to the effects of the high levels of circulating insulin, the only way that our bodies can compensate is to produce *even more insulin*! This is the condition called 'hyperinsulinism' – or, more simply, far too much insulin.

As the insulin levels increase, eventually the pancreas cannot make enough insulin for the needs of our body and we develop diabetes, which has to be treated by diet, oral medication or even more insulin by injection.

The main complications of diabetes are heart disease, damage to the nervous system, kidney failure and blindness. In fact, diabetes is the commonest cause of blindness in those under 65 in the United Kingdom. And all of these dreadful effects are the direct consequence of a disease which, in many cases, results from a diet based on refined carbohydrates!

Let us summarise the problem:

- Insulin is a hormone which has effects on every cell in the body.
- Insulin is absolutely essential for health but too much insulin is detrimental to health.
- Carbohydrates are the main stimulus for insulin production.
- Too much carbohydrate causes the production of too much insulin.

And the consequences of overproduction of insulin (hyper-insulinism) are increased risk of:

- Obesity
- Heart disease
- High blood pressure
- Arthritis (due to obesity)
- Diabetes
- Kidney failure (secondary to diabetes)
- Visual problems (possibly leading to blindness) as a result of diabetes

Insulin levels cannot be lowered by medication. They can only be lowered by alteration of diet, which is common sense as the problem is caused by excess carbohydrates in our diet.

The obvious solution to the problem of overproduction of insulin is to reduce the production of insulin by *reducing carbohydrates in our diet*. To ensure weight loss – but at the same time preventing malnutrition from vitamin and mineral deficiencies –

you have to reduce your carbohydrate intake to approximately 40–50 grams per day. There are excellent carbohydrate counters to guide you (such as *The Ultimate Diet Counter*) but as a generalisation one slice of bread contains 15–17 grams of carbohydrate and an egg contains no carbohydrate!

The obvious next question is which foods contain refined carbohydrates and should therefore be avoided. The answer is complicated by the fact that there are 'natural' carbohydrates associated with vegetables and fruit that we include in the diet in moderation, whilst processed, 'refined' carbohydrates (such as white bread, cakes and confectionery) must be completely excluded. The differences between 'healthy' unrefined carbohydrates and 'unhealthy' refined carbohydrates will be discussed in the next chapter; however, in simple terms, foods may be categorised as follows:

## Virtually no-carb foods

- All animal-based products, including beef, pork, lamb and poultry
- All fish and shellfish
- Eggs
- Cheese
- All 'pure' fats, including oils (such as olive oil) and butter
- Herbs
- Spices
- Low-calorie soft drinks
- Tea
- Artificial sweeteners
- Alcoholic spirits (whisky, gin, brandy)

## Medium-carb foods

- Most vegetables (except potatoes, parsnips and – to a lesser extent – carrots)
- Most fruits (except banana, mango and pineapple)
- Dairy products (milk, yoghurt, cream)
- Fruit juices
- Pulses (peas, beans, lentils)
- Red wine and dry white wine

## High-carb foods

- Bread
- Rice
- Pasta
- All cakes, confectionery, sweets and biscuits
- All pies and pastries
- Flour
- Root vegetables (potatoes, parsnips)
- All cereals (including breakfast cereals)
- Beer, cider, sweet white wine, fortified wines (sherry, port)

Never reduce your carbohydrate intake below 40–50 grams per day as to do so will mean that you are restricting vegetables from your diet, and that will inevitably lead to nutritional deficiencies. The only, less desirable, alternative is to take multivitamin supplements, but if you keep to the level of 40–50 grams of unrefined carbohydrates, that will not be necessary.

However this diet is not simply based on the carbohydrate content of foods. On the contrary, it takes into account many other relevant factors, such as the Glycaemic Index of foods (Chapter 4) and the insulinogenic effect of some foods (see over).

The essential problem with providing a perfect diet for every individual is that each and every person is intrinsically unique. This seems obvious, but it has very serious medical (and therefore dietary) implications. For example, one person may have a high insulin level whilst another may be lower. One individual may be grossly overweight whilst another may be only slightly overweight. In each and every case the response to a diet which is *medically based* will obviously be different – because the individuals have different medical characteristics at the commencement of the diet.

Similarly, the effect of carbohydrates on stimulating insulin production does not follow the simple rules one would expect in every case. For example, in some individuals, dairy products produce a far higher insulin response than their carbohydrate content would merit. This means that the insulin response is higher than expected and the weight loss is therefore lower than would be anticipated on the basis of the carb content alone.

In other words, there are many other factors to be taken into account than simply the carb content of foods in a low-carb diet.

This diet has taken into consideration all of the known medical factors to ensure healthy weight loss; all you have to do is follow the simple principles described in Chapter 7 to enjoy a successful diet.

# Chapter **3** Low-carb diets – the myths exposed

In essence, a diet which restricts refined carbohydrates is basically healthy. Refined carbohydrates have no intrinsic nutritional value whatsoever and only have any value at all as a result of the additives, which are required by law simply because governments realised the health risks of a diet based on refined carbohydrates without these additives.

But note that it is only **refined** carbohydrates that are unhealthy: white bread, refined pasta, polished rice, confectionery, cakes and pastry in all forms. **Unrefined** carbohydrates are healthy – those in natural products such as vegetables, fruit, pulses, dairy products and wholegrains. Unfortunately, our bodies cannot differentiate between 'good' unrefined carbohydrates and 'bad' refined carbohydrates, so we must *restrict* – not exclude – the 'good' carbohydrates whilst dieting. Diets which restrict *all* carbohydrates can be potentially dangerous unless nutritional supplements are taken.

Surely a diet based on low carbohydrates must be high in fats – or so many nutritionists would have us believe. Nonsense! There is absolutely no requirement for a high fat intake on a low-carb diet. A certain amount of 'pure' fats must be included in a healthy diet as we require some of the 'good' fats in order to absorb vitamins A, D, E and K, which are absolutely essential; these are fat-soluble vitamins, which means that if you have a diet very low in fats you cannot absorb these nutrients and malnutrition is an inevitable consequence.

As you will see from this diet, there is relatively little fat included and it is a low-carbohydrate diet that excludes red meat. Dairy products and eggs are included, in moderation, also fish and shellfish; however, they can be excluded from the diet for vegetarians. It is not essential to eat fish and shellfish to be healthy, but they are such nutritious (and delicious) foods that we would strongly advise you to include them in your diet unless you have moral beliefs to the contrary.

This book has been produced in response to the immense number of requests we have received from many different sources for a low-carbohydrate diet that excludes meat, and is therefore low in saturated fats. Many individuals have chosen to avoid animal products for a variety of very understandable reasons, not just for reasons of health but also on grounds of morality. It has often been stated that low-carb diets are based on meat and therefore cannot be applied to vegetarians, and this has been used as one of the most forceful arguments against a low-carb diet. In fact, nothing is further from the truth – yet another myth put forward by those who are so adamantly opposed to the low-carb diet.

Another frequent (and equally inaccurate) criticism of low-carb diets by certain ill-informed commentators is that they are unhealthy because they don't contain pasta, rice, grains and pulses. This is similarly nonsense! If a low-carb diet is nutritionally balanced (as *The New High Protein Diet* certainly is) it will include all of the essential nutrients which are present in those foods; there are no nutritional essentials in grains and pulses that are not present in other foods.

However, many individuals would like to include these nutritious foods in their diet and this system proves categorically that there is absolutely no reason why this cannot be achieved. In this modification of our diet, we have omitted meat and included wholemeal rice, wholemeal pasta and wholemeal bread, plus fruits and pulses, in moderation.

So apart from those carbohydrate addicts who simply cannot live without their high-carbohydrate foods, this diet proves conclusively that everyone, whatever their dietary preference, can enjoy a low-carb lifestyle and the health benefits which will inevitably follow.

The reason why animal products are included in our original low-carb diet (*The New High Protein Diet*, published by Vermilion) is that foods of animal origin contain all the essential amino acids that we require for the building of body proteins. So including foods of animal origin is the easiest way to obtain these essential nutrients, effectively without any effort or pre-planning.

But that is not to say that one cannot obtain all of the essential amino acids from foods of plant origin – of course this is possible, as evidenced by the large population of very healthy vegetarians! It simply involves a little more planning and forethought because, apart from tofu, no food of plant origin contains *all* of the essential amino acids for health. Including both grains and pulses in a vegetarian diet will ensure the inclusion of all essential amino acids, which are required to manufacture body proteins. Of course, if you include dairy products, eggs (and/or fish and shellfish) then the problem is solved as these contain all essential amino acids.

So whether you are a vegetarian or simply someone who has decided to forego eating meat, it is equally simple to enjoy the healthy advantages of a low-carb diet which excludes refined carbohydrates.

Low-carbohydrate diets are here to stay, despite the most strenuous efforts of so-called experts who assure us that they are not safe. They omit to provide one single shred of evidence for this absurd statement and dismiss the scientific evidence to date which clearly shows that diets low in refined carbohydrates are much healthier than those simply low in fats or calories. The rationale of low-carbohydrate dieting is explained in Chapter 1, but the scientific evidence is irrefutable – the simple fact is that it works (unlike low-calorie diets in 95 per cent of cases).

# Chapter 4    Glycaemic Index – the key to low-carb success

The Glycaemic Index – or GI – seems just another complicated factor for the dedicated dieter to consider. But is it? Actually no – it is a very simple concept embodied within the principles of a diet low in refined carbohydrates.

Basically the GI is a measure of the effects of any particular food on blood glucose levels over a period of time. Sounds complicated, but as with virtually everything in medicine it is actually very simple. The standard against which all foods are compared is the absorption of glucose and its effects on blood glucose levels over a period of several hours. Glucose is rapidly absorbed from the gut into the bloodstream. Other foods – almost, but not completely, without exception – are absorbed more slowly and have a lesser effect on the rate of increase of blood glucose levels. The Glycaemic Index is quite simply a measure of the effects of any other food in elevating blood sugar (glucose) levels compared to glucose. To simplify the comparison, glucose has been arbitrarily assigned the figure of 100 and all other foods are therefore a percentage of this effect on raising blood sugar levels. For example, a high-GI food such as bread has a GI of 70 and therefore will increase blood sugar levels at about 70 per cent of the rate of pure glucose, but a food with a low-GI value – such as chickpeas – has only 28 per cent of the effect of glucose on raising blood sugar levels.

And, of course, foods that contain virtually no carbohydrates (such as meat, fish, eggs, poultry, cheese, cream, olive oil, avocado, mayonnaise, most nuts and shellfish) have virtually no effect on blood sugar levels and therefore have a GI of zero! Foods with a very low carbohydrate content – which includes most fresh vegetables – also have a very low GI.

In summary, the foods included (virtually without restriction) in a diet low in refined carbohydrates are also low-GI foods. In other words, their capacity to increase blood glucose levels is low or negligible.

What is the relevance of a low-GI/low-carb diet to health? Quite simply a low-carb diet is, by definition, low-GI. This means that the stimulation of insulin from blood sugar is low and therefore insulin levels are low. As insulin is the main hormone controlling the production of fat cells – and actively preventing the breakdown of fat cells – a diet low in refined carbohydrates is essentially a low-GI diet: they are one and the same entity, producing the same beneficial effect on health – the reduction of insulin.

It is, however, essential to distinguish between a generalised *low-carb diet* and a diet *low in refined carbohydrates*. The former restricts *all* carbohydrates, including those which are slowly absorbed (i.e. low-GI) and therefore have a lesser capacity to stimulate insulin release. Many current low-carb diets reduce *all* carbohydrates in the diet, irrespective of whether they are *refined* carbohydrates (and therefore of little nutritional value) or *unrefined* carbohydrates (and therefore of essential nutritional value). If this means reducing natural carbohydrate foods, which include other essential vitamins and minerals (such as vegetables), this may have serious deleterious effects on health unless vitamin and mineral supplements are included in the form of tablets – we do not advocate this approach.

On the other hand, the diet we advocate, restricting only *refined* carbohydrates (bread, pasta, rice, cakes, sweets), with lesser restrictions on the more healthy higher-carb foods (pulses, fruit and milk) and virtually no restrictions on vegetables, ensures that the diet contains *all* of the essential nutrition for health, and is still very successful as a low-GI/low-carb diet.

The *natural* carbohydrates found in vegetables are inextricably linked to the essential vitamins and minerals present in vegetables.

Because vegetables have a low GI and include many essential nutrients for health, these should not be restricted in a healthy diet – and, more importantly, you can see that because these have a low GI there is no need to restrict these foods in a successful low-carb diet because they have a much lesser capacity to stimulate insulin production.

In other words, it is very simple to follow a diet which has the dual advantages of being both low-carb and low-GI as both are complementary attributes to a healthy diet.

In our view, all essential nutrition can – and should – be provided by natural sources from the diet: poultry, fish, shellfish, eggs, cheese, pulses, natural essential oils and vegetables. The basis of this diet is the provision of all essential nutrients, naturally.

However, the issue is slightly more complex as some foods may have similar quantities of carbohydrates but different rates of absorption. For example, pasta and rice contain similar proportions of carbohydrates (at about 70 per cent) but the Glycaemic Index of rice is high (at 83) whilst the Glycaemic Index of pasta is lower than expected at 40–50. This is simply explained by the fact that pasta is absorbed more slowly than rice. The *relevance* and *importance* is that the slower absorption of pasta means that it stimulates a lesser response of insulin and therefore has a lesser capacity to stimulate fat production.

This means that we *can* include pasta in this diet, in restricted quantities, because it is absorbed at a lesser rate. Rice is also included in the diet, but in much lower quantities because of its greater capacity to stimulate insulin (and therefore fat production).

This is further complicated by the fact that different forms of rice have different rates of absorption (and different GI); for example, Arborio rice has a much lower GI (at 58) than Jasmine rice (at 109). So obviously we have included Arborio rice in this low-GI/low-carb diet as it has the lowest Glycaemic Index of the rice family; it is therefore absorbed more slowly and has a lesser effect on the stimulation of insulin.

You don't need to know the GI values of different foods. All of the variables have been factored into this diet. However, it is important that you understand the medical basis of the diet and the reasons *why* you are following this programme.

In essence, the key to successful weight loss is lowering insulin resistance and therefore reducing circulating levels of insulin. This is achieved by reducing daily carbohydrate intake to 40–50 grams per day, primarily by the reduction of refined carbohydrates. If refined carbohydrates are included in the diet, they must be restricted within the 40–50 gram limit, preferably including those with a low GI (and therefore a lower capacity to stimulate insulin production).

And any healthy diet must include all of the essential amino acids, essential fatty acids, vitamins and minerals for continued health.

This diet, low in refined carbohydrates and incorporating mainly foods with a low Glycaemic Index, has been carefully designed to incorporate all of the essential nutrition, and is successful in both achieving sustainable weight loss and at the same time maintaining optimal nutrition for health.

# Chapter 5 Health benefits of a low-GI/low-carb diet

Having explained *why* a diet low in refined carbohydrates is healthy, it is now essential to explain the medical rationale for this statement. And we will proceed to *prove* these assertions by medical evidence from actual case studies.

We have treated many patients with weight problems in our clinics in London and Edinburgh. Every patient is medically different and each has specific personal idiosyncrasies which must be incorporated into their diet. That is the essential problem in trying to formulate our experiences in a single book – or even a series of books. When an overweight patient attends a physician in clinic, it is relatively straightforward to identify the problems with their diet and to design an appropriate dietary plan.

In a proportion of cases, there is obviously an underlying medical problem which requires treatment. However, in virtually every situation, the overweight patient has hyperinsulinism – too much insulin as a direct result of a diet with a high proportion of refined carbohydrates. In other words, *the patient has a medical problem*. They are not overweight merely because they have been overeating (although that may be the case), but rather because the type of food in their diet is causing hyperinsulinism. They have been consuming a diet high in carbohydrates, stimulating the production of too much insulin, which causes fat deposition.

Before describing the cases in detail, it would be useful to explain the meaning of a few simple medical terms (which many experienced dieters will already understand) and which are central to understanding the weight problem – and its solution.

## Body Mass Index

Body Mass Index (BMI) is a measure of how over- or under-weight we are compared to our height. In seemingly complicated terms, it is calculated by the weight (in kilograms) divided by the height (in centimetres) squared! In simple terms, normal is between 20–25, overweight is 25–30 and obese is over 30. Seems complicated but is really very simple.

## Insulin

Insulin is the hormone which controls fat production and prevents fat breakdown. The normal fasting level would be less than 10 mIU/l; increased levels are indicative of hyper-insulinism. Once again, in simple terms, if you have elevated levels of insulin *it is virtually impossible to break down body fat – irrespective of the number of calories in your diet*. Insulin controls the deposition of body fat and the breakdown of body fat. If the insulin level is high (as a result of too many refined carbohydrates in the diet) *then you cannot break down the fat*.

As the insulin levels are increased to unacceptable levels by stimulation from a high-carb diet, eventually the pancreas cannot produce any more and this is the disease called type 2 diabetes. If you reduce your need for insulin by reducing refined carbohydrates, the risks of developing acquired diabetes decreases exponentially.

Even worse, insulin stimulates the production of Low Density Lipoproteins (LDL), which are the 'bad' forms of cholesterol in our blood. These promote the deposition of cholesterol in our arteries leading to heart disease. The many other adverse consequences of a high insulin level (hyperinsulinism) are explained in Chapter 2.

**A diet low in refined carbohydrates lowers insulin levels, reducing the risk of heart disease and diabetes.**

# Triglycerides

Serum triglycerides are fats in the blood which are a serious factor in the development of heart disease. As with all of these various blood parameters, they must be measured after a 12-hour fast. The normal level is less than 2.3 mmol/l, but these are usually significantly elevated in patients with raised insulin levels.

# Cholesterol

Cholesterol is difficult to measure in itself because the level of cholesterol in the blood actually includes several different types of cholesterol. In simple terms, there are 'good' cholesterols and 'bad' cholesterols. What does this mean? Surely all cholesterol in the blood is a serious indicator of heart disease. Not so! In fact, nothing could be further from the truth.

## High Density Lipoproteins (HDL)

HDL (or high density lipoprotein) is a good form of cholesterol which transports the fatty deposits *away* from the arteries and therefore protects against heart disease. These are usually **low** in hyperinsulinism, which is dangerous to health.

## Low Density Lipoproteins (LDL)

LDL (or low density lipoprotein) is a bad form of cholesterol which deposits blood fats in the arteries and therefore promotes heart disease. This is usually **high** in hyperinsulinism, which once again is very undesirable.

So you can easily see that a measure of cholesterol by itself is meaningless. If the cholesterol level is high, it may be due to high HDL (which is good) or high LDL (which is bad). You must have a breakdown of the type of cholesterol for this to be a meaningful measure.

Of course, this is a very simplified version of the many different sub-types that constitute the level of fats in the blood, but it provides an effective guideline by which everyone can easily understand the importance of different fats in the blood, and, more importantly, the advantageous effects of a diet low in refined carbohydrates on the blood lipid profile.

## Case studies

Having described the immense beneficial effects of a diet low in refined carbohydrates on health, it is necessary to substantiate these assertions by verifiable evidence, the most reliable source being actual case studies. Biochemical parameters provide *objective* evidence for the advantages of medical treatment. And there should be no doubt whatsoever that the improvement of health by manipulation of diet is a very potent medical treatment – without the potential side-effects of drugs or surgery.

All of these parameters (and others where indicated) are measured on all of our patients undergoing weight-loss management in our clinics. The following case histories demonstrate how important it is to measure these parameters in patients with weight problems, and how they can be normalised by appropriate diet. We have specifically described the series of health changes that occurred in the first four-week period of the diet in all cases in order that equivalent comparisons can be made, and also to demonstrate that significant improvements in both weight and the blood parameters can be achieved in a relatively brief period of time.

A selection of widely disparate patients with different lifestyles and different medical problems has been deliberately chosen to illustrate the medical advantages of this diet. Some are simply overweight and need to diet; others have early or severe diabetes; and others have both severe diabetes and severe heart disease. The only common factor among all of these patients is that all derived considerable medical benefits from following a diet low in refined carbohydrates. All of them had been following different low-calorie diets for many years. All were highly motivated and all had been singularly unsuccessful in losing weight!

Their high-carbohydrate diets had caused hyperinsulinism, which in turn prevented them from breaking down their body fat no matter how devoutly they adhered to their former low-calorie dietary regime.

## Case 1

Mr A is a 29-year-old grocer in a major city. His lifestyle is hectic and busy. He rises at 5 a.m. to attend the fruit and vegetable market each weekday, then spends the rest of the morning delivering produce to various retail outlets. His first meal of the day is 11.30 a.m., usually a sandwich followed by (not surprisingly) several pieces of fruit. A busy afternoon is followed by a take-away meal in the evening, often Indian or Chinese. He drinks moderately, but always beer.

He weighed 94.9 kg, which equates to a BMI of 38 when height is taken into account, and is obviously overweight.

This patient has a hectic lifestyle which is dictated by the requirements of his occupation. He has no apparent time to eat a balanced diet evenly distributed throughout the day. We convinced the patient of the absolute necessity of making time for a substantial breakfast low in refined carbohydrates for two reasons; to provide a slow release of energy gradually throughout the morning and to prevent the production of insulin by reducing the carbohydrate content.

After four weeks on the diet, his weight had reduced to 90.3 kg, with a reduction of BMI to 34.8. Of much more significance was the fact that fasting serum triglycerides reduced by 17 per cent from 0.98 mmol/l to 0.82 mmol/l and fasting serum HDL increased by 11 per cent from 1.05 mmol/l to 1.17 mmol/l.

### Comment

This patient had a serious lifestyle problem causing obesity. By changing his eating habits, making time for breakfast, transferring to a diet high in protein and low in refined carbohydrates, he was able to achieve sustained weight loss and significant improvements in his blood lipid parameters, reducing triglycerides (which are 'bad' for the heart) and increasing HDL (which is 'good' for the heart).

## Case 2

This young lady is a 27-year-old secretary with a significant weight problem since early childhood. Most of her immediate family were overweight and she had assumed that this was a genetic feature of the family. She had tried virtually every form of diet over the previous 15 years, obviously without success. Her total calorie intake was not excessively high but the diet was extremely low fat, consisting of approximately 75 per cent carbohydrate and the remainder protein, with virtually no fat in the diet.

With an initial weight of 128.9 kg and height of 163.2 cm, this equated to a BMI of 49 – considerably in excess of the obesity limit of 30! Total cholesterol level was high at 5.9 mmol/l, which was primarily caused by the high level of the dangerous LDL at 4.06 mmol/l.

After one month conscientiously adhering to the diet her weight had reduced to 121.8 kg, a reduction of 7.1 kg. Total cholesterol had reduced to 4.9 mmol/l, a reduction of 17 per cent, but of much more significance was the fact that this was entirely due to a reduction in LDL by 23 per cent from 4.06 to 3.11 mmol/l. HDL, the cholesterol which is protective to the heart, had actually increased from 1.44 to 1.49 mmol/l, and triglycerides, which are particularly dangerous blood lipids, had reduced from 0.99 mmol/l to 0.79 mmol/l, once again an incredible reduction of 20 per cent.

## Comment

This young woman was at considerable risk of all the medical complications of obesity in later life. Almost certainly there will have been some irreversible arthritic changes in both the hip and knee joints as a consequence of 15 years of considerable stress from excess weight. The risk of heart disease was already present, with increased total cholesterol consisting of increased levels of the dangerous LDL. These problems were immediately addressed by significant reductions in weight, total cholesterol, LDL and triglycerides, with an associated increase in HDL.

## Case 3

This patient is a 61-year-old self-employed businessman with a significant past medical history of type 2 diabetes for 10 years and two episodes of quadruple coronary bypass surgery in that period, the most recent surgery within the past year.

His initial weight was 99.6 kg which equated to a BMI of 35. Fasting insulin level was 49.7 mIU/l, confirming the presence of insulin resistance (the normal level is less than 10). His fasting glucose level was high at 10.9 mmol/l (the normal is less than 6 mmol/l).

Of much more significance was the triglyceride level of 5.69 mmol/l. Triglycerides are one of the most significant risk factors for heart disease. This patient's level is 2.4 times the highest acceptable level and he was at extreme risk as he had already undergone quadruple bypass surgery on two previous occasions. His HDL was low at 1.04 mmol/l and LDL ratio could not be calculated because the triglyceride level was too high for the calculation to be made!

After one month on the diet his weight had reduced by almost 6 kg to 93.7 kg. Blood parameters had improved phenomenally. Triglycerides had reduced to 2.86 mmol/l, a reduction of 50 per cent, and this reduced even further a month later to 1.45 mmol/l. This represents a reduction in triglyceride levels by 75 per cent in two months and now well within normal limits. There was an associated increase in the protective HDL from 1.04 mmol/l to 1.34 mmol/l in the same period, an increase of 29 per cent. Total cholesterol reduced from 4.9 mmol/l to 4.0 mmol/l (18 per cent) which is obviously due to LDL as the protective HDL had increased by 20 per cent in that period.

Fasting insulin level reduced by 62 per cent from 49.7 mIU/l to 18.9 mIU/l. As the lipid levels are primarily controlled by the insulin level, this reduction is the ultimate reason for the significant lowering of triglycerides and increase in HDL cholesterol.

### Comment

It would be no exaggeration to state that this diet had significantly improved this patient's diabetic control and cardiovascular health. He had already undergone quadruple coronary bypass surgery twice and was at considerable risk of continuing heart problems with triglyceride levels almost 2.5 times the upper limit of normal. Total cholesterol was significantly elevated.

Within two months, triglyceride levels had reduced by 75 per cent, cholesterol had reduced by 18 per cent and the HDL level (which is protective to the heart) had increased by 29 per cent. Diabetic control was improved dramatically by a reduction of the fasting insulin level by 62 per cent, which permitted reduction in medications required to control diabetes.

## Case 4

This patient is a 31-year-old office worker with weight problems of more than 20 years. Once again, most of the other family members were significantly overweight so it was considered by the family to be possibly a genetic problem. He had been dieting intermittently for over 15 years without success.

Initial weight was 116.8 kg which, in conjunction with a height of 186.7 cm, gave a BMI of 34. After four weeks his weight had reduced by 5.9 kg to 110.9 kg, with a further reduction to 108.5 kg a month later. Over the same period, triglyceride levels reduced by 16 per cent from 1.13 mmol/l to 0.95 mmol/l. This continued to decrease and six months later the level was 0.62 mmol/l, an incredible reduction of 45 per cent.

Similar trends were demonstrated by fasting cholesterol levels. Total cholesterol reduced from 6.0 mmol/l to 5.8 mmol/l in the first month, with continuing reductions to 4.4 mmol/l after six months, a decrease of almost 17 per cent. This was entirely as a result of reduction in LDL levels, from 4.7 to 3.03 (36 per cent); HDL levels increased by 35 per cent from 0.80 to 1.08 mmol/l. Over the same period, fasting insulin levels continued to fall from an initial level of 28.2 mlU/l to 15.4 mlU/l.

## Comment

This is a typical history of a young man with significant weight problems entirely as a result of inappropriate and frankly absurd dietary advice. This patient, as many others, had been con-scientiously following dietary advice based upon a low-fat, high-carbohydrate regime that was not only guaranteed to produce no significant weight loss, but actually the opposite! On a nutritionally balanced diet low in refined carbohydrates, he utilised body fat, lost weight and substantially improved blood lipid levels at a stroke. He improved his personal appearance and significantly reduced his subsequent risk of heart disease by reducing LDL levels by 36 per cent and increasing HDL levels by 35 per cent.

## Case 5

This 52-year-old lady who had a 'mild' weight problem: at 78.3 kg and a height of 157.9 cm, the BMI was 31, just over the accepted obesity limit of 30. The patient had a supposedly 'healthy' carbohydrate-based diet, which means that it consisted of many carbs said by many nutritionists to be 'healthy' (such as pasta and rice) but actually very unhealthy. The patient had a particular problem as she travelled extensively by air – and everyone on a low-carb diet is aware of the problems with airline cuisine!

Once again, as so often is the case with patients following the regime of a 'healthy' carbohydrate-based diet, the blood lipid profile was abysmal! Fasting triglyceride levels were excessively elevated at 5.02 mmol/l, fasting total cholesterol was similarly excessive at 5.60 mmol/l and HDL was low at 0.96 mmol/l. LDL levels could not be estimated because of the very high triglyceride levels!

After four weeks her weight had reduced by 3.1 kg to 75.2 kg. One month later this had reduced to 73.7 kg. Fasting triglyceride levels had reduced by 52 per cent to 2.41 mmol/l. Fasting total cholesterol had reduced by 20 per cent to 4.5 mmol/l and HDL had increased by 22 per cent to 1.17 mmol/l – with the inevitable conclusion that the reduction in total cholesterol was as a result of reduction in LDL. Fasting insulin levels reduced by 36 per cent from 6.1 mIU/l to 3.9 mIU/l.

### Comment

This patient had significant weight reduction on this form of low-GI/low-carb diet. Triglyceride levels reduced by an incredible 52 per cent in one month, HDL increased by 22 per cent and total cholesterol reduced by 20 per cent – all contributing to a significantly reduced risk of subsequent heart disease.

## Case 6

This patient is a 65-year-old businessman with a long history of dieting unsuccessfully. He exercised regularly and had conscientiously followed strict dietary advice on a low-fat, low-calorie diet – and failed to lose weight. He had a long history of type 2 diabetes controlled by oral medication, but his insulin level remained high at 25.1 mIU/l indicating significant insulin resistance.

An initial weight of 119.2 kg with a height of 195 cm gave a BMI of 31. Four weeks later his weight had reduced by 2.6 kg to 116.6 kg. Weight loss continued at a steady rate over the succeeding two months with the loss of a further 3.1 kg. There was also an associated significant improvement in the blood lipids. Triglycerides reduced by 42 per cent from 1.16 mmol/l to 0.67 mmol/l. LDL reduced by 17 per cent from 1.57 mmol/l to 1.30 mmol/l and HDL increased by 22 per cent from 1.13 mmol/l to 1.38 mmol/l. His energy levels improved exponentially and body shape changed dramatically, as a result of replacing fat with muscle.

### Comment

As has been stated on several occasions in this (and previous) books, weight loss is virtually impossible in the presence of a high insulin levels. This patient's low-carb diet reduced insulin levels to normal at 8.2 mIU/l within one month, diabetic control improved and oral diabetic medications were reduced. The risk of heart disease was substantially reduced by the significant reductions in triglycerides and LDL, with the associated increase in HDL.

## Case 7

This was a long-standing diabetic patient, a 54-year-old, highly intelligent teacher who had carefully followed the carbohydrate-based diet he had been prescribed by a nutritionist and whose diabetes had subsequently been very difficult to control.

His initial weight was 99.7 kg with a BMI of 30. Initial fasting insulin levels were high at 27.9 mlU/l. Total cholesterol was elevated at 5.7 mmol/l and triglycerides were high at 3.9 mmol/l.

One month after commencing the diet there had been a reduction of 2 kg in weight to 97.7 kg. Insulin levels had reduced by 44 per cent to 15.6 mlU/l. Total cholesterol reduced by 32 per cent to 3.9 mmol/l, triglycerides reduced by 55 per cent to 1.74 mmol/l, LDL reduced by 30 per cent from 2.85 mmol/l to 2.0 mmol/l and HDL increased by 15 per cent from 1.04 mmol/l to 1.20 mmol/l.

### Comment

As a result of the diet, control of diabetes was significantly improved, diabetic medication was reduced and the risks of heart disease from elevated blood lipids virtually eliminated. The patient has more energy and feels better subjectively. More importantly, he is much less worried about his health because he can see objective measures of improvement in both his diabetic control and blood lipids for the first time. Previously, he believed that deterioration was inevitable because the results always seemed to worsen despite all of his best efforts to follow the previous high-carb-based dietary advice he had been given.

## Conclusions

What can we conclude from these typical examples of the effects of a diet low in refined carbohydrates?

After a month on this diet, there was an average reduction in weight of 4.4 kg. Total cholesterol reduced by an average of 21 per cent, but this was totally as a result of the reduction in 'bad' cholesterol, as LDL levels reduced by an average of 26 per cent whilst the 'good' HDL levels increased by 22 per cent. Of much greater significance is the fact that the dangerous triglyceride levels reduced by an average of 40 per cent. The effects on fasting insulin levels are similarly dramatic with an average reduction of 48 per cent in four weeks.

Objective measurement of blood parameters therefore demonstrate significant health benefits of a diet low in refined carbohydrates. In each of these patients, the results continued to improve or stabilise over the succeeding six months. No patient on the programme experienced any reversal of results.

**However it is important to emphasise that no diet is perfect for everyone.** As stated previously, we are all very different individuals with different medical characteristics. A low-GI/low-carb diet has been clearly shown to be very successful in achieving sustainable weight loss and with significant health benefits, but this is entirely dependent upon the pre-existing medical health of the individual. As a generalisation, we would strongly advise everyone contemplating *any* diet to check with their physician first. In our clinics we treat obesity as a serious disease – which it is – and all patients are carefully monitored throughout the dietary programme. This is desirable, but not absolutely essential, for successful dieting in most individuals, but it is essential in those with pre-existing medical conditions.

## Calcium and osteoporosis

One final health note on health. Some of the detractors of high-protein diets have made statements to the effect that they cause loss of calcium and will therefore lead to osteoporosis. There is no medical evidence for this assertion. For example, in the patients quoted there was no significant difference between the blood calcium levels at the commencement of the diet and one month later.

We routinely measure blood calcium levels in all of our patients and calcium levels remain stable on the diet. In other words, there is no evidence that a high-protein diet causes loss of calcium; on the contrary, the evidence clearly shows a stable calcium level on this diet, which is hardly surprising as our diet includes the foods which are particularly high in calcium levels: dairy produce and fatty fish. Incidentally these are the foods which are usually severely restricted on a typical low-fat/low-calorie diet!

Another myth exposed.

# Chapter **6** Essential nutrients for health

You don't *need* to read this chapter!

Our guiding principle throughout the series of lifestyle books we have published is to promote health through the most effective dietary means possible, in association with practical forms of exercise – walking and isometrics rather than gymnastic Olympian efforts! This chapter has only been included to explain to those interested that all of the essential nutrients that we require for health are included in abundance in this diet. This is based on objective medical evidence. There are no unsubstantiated medical claims.

Some dietitians and nutritionists seem to consider their life's aim to be to denigrate low-carb diets in general. I would entirely agree that there are some low-carb diets which are not nutritionally balanced, just as there are many low-calorie diets which are not nutritionally balanced – but this diet is balanced and contains all of the essential vitamins, minerals, amino acids and essential fatty acids for health.

More importantly, medical studies (as described in Chapter 5) have proved the health advantages of this diet in weight reduction, risk of diabetes, risk of heart disease and reducing high blood pressure.

A diet must be nutritionally safe – in other words, it *must* include all of the essential nutrients for health. Unfortunately, many diets are not safe. For example, a typical low-calorie diet requires the individual to consume fewer calories (as food) than they require. Obviously, this means fewer nutrients, and unless you are very careful malnourishment is an inevitable result! It certainly is not necessary for you to learn all of the essential nutrients for health, but it is essential that you are convinced that you will obtain all of the essential nutrition from any diet. Interestingly, very few diet books provide that information, presumably because very few diets actually provide all of the nutrition you need – in other words, the diets are actually making you unwell!

This diet is different. Whilst it is quite simple to obtain all of the essential nutrients on a diet including foods of animal origin, it is also relatively simple to do so on a typical vegetarian diet, whilst excluding refined carbohydrates. Refined carbohydrates (white rice, pasta, bread and sugars) *provide no nutrition whatsoever* (without added nutrients), but are merely sources of energy – which can be equally provided by essential proteins and fats. Refined carbohydrates have no intrinsic vitamins or minerals; in fact they are so devoid of any nutrients in their natural state that vitamins and minerals are added because the government has legislated that these nutrients must be included!

In order that you can be absolutely certain you are obtaining all of the essential nutrients for health from your diet, here is a brief list of the most essential proteins, fatty acids, vitamins and minerals. Obviously, it is not possible to include all essential nutrients in a book of this nature – and it isn't necessary because you can be certain that they will be included in the diet. You don't need to remember any of this list: it is included merely to demonstrate that all of the essential nutrients are present in abundance in the foods included in this diet.

Of course, there are many essential nutrients in red meat, but as this has been excluded from the diet we have not described the nutrients from meat-based products in the following list.

## Essential amino acids

What are 'amino acids' and why are they so essential? Amino acids are commonly called the 'building blocks of life' because they combine to form the body proteins that make up the structure of the body. There are 22 amino acids, 13 of which can be made by our bodies, the remaining nine being considered 'essential' as they must be supplied from the diet. Only three of these 'essential' amino acids cause a problem in a vegetarian-based diet, as the others are commonly found in many foods of plant origin. The three which are found primarily in specific groups of plant foods in different proportions are known as methionine, lysine and tryptophan. Grain-based products (such as wholegrains) are excellent sources of methionine and tryptophan, whilst pulses (such as peas or beans) are rich in lysine. Is it essential to understand these complex medical issues? Certainly not! But it is essential that you understand the basis for including certain foods in a vegetarian-based diet, as all vegetables do not contain all of the essential amino acids for life – unlike animal-based products.

So if you combine grains and pulses you will satisfy all of your amino acid requirements. Unfortunately, these foods are also relatively high in carbohydrate content, but they can still be included in a low-carb diet in moderation. And as soya and its many derivatives (such as tofu) is a 'complete' protein which contains all essential amino acids, you can always be certain of avoiding amino acid deficiencies in your diet by including this delicious and nutritious ingredient.

Of course, many people are not strictly vegetarian, but have rather decided to exclude meat products from their diet. In this case there is really no problem as fish, shellfish, eggs and dairy products (milk and cheese) are 'complete' proteins which contain all of the essential amino acids.

## Essential fatty acids

There are some fats which you require for health – not the ubiquitous hydrogenated fats present in pastries and confectionery, but omega-3 and omega-6 fatty acids.

## Omega-3 fatty acids

The richest source of these essential nutrients is undoubtedly the so-called 'fatty fish', such as mackerel, herrings, sardines, salmon and tuna, but they are also present in soya, beans, wholegrains, eggs, certain seeds (for example, flaxseed), nuts and seaweed. The vegetable purslane is a particularly rich source of omega-3 fatty acids.

## Omega-6 fatty acids

The best source is seeds and their oils (especially sunflower, safflower and sesame), wholegrains, soya beans, some vegetables and eggs.

# Vitamins

Vitamins are chemicals which are found in minute quantities in many natural foods, which are essential for health. Most processed foods are very poor sources of vitamins.

## Vitamin A

This vitamin is present in many fruits and vegetables, particularly carrots, red peppers, tomatoes, spinach and mangetout. It is also present in fish, eggs, butter and cheese.

## Vitamin B$^1$

Vitamin B$^1$ is present in Quorn$^{TM}$ mycoprotein, nuts (especially Brazils, peanuts and pine nuts), sesame seeds, sunflower seeds, tahini and fish – particularly salmon.

## Vitamin B$^2$

Present in mushrooms, avocados, almonds and wheat germ, as well as fish, shellfish, cheese and eggs.

## Vitamin B$^3$
Excellent sources of niacin are wheat bran, nuts, sesame seeds, sunflower seeds and tahini. Non-plant sources include tuna, mackerel, salmon, trout, cheese and eggs.

## Vitamin B$^6$ (Pyridoxine)
Present in wheat germ, wheat bran, sesame seeds, nuts (especially walnuts, hazelnuts and peanuts), garlic, avocados, tomatoes and tomato purée. Pyridoxine is also present in many fish (especially salmon, tuna, mackerel and haddock).

## Vitamin B$^{12}$
This is the only vitamin not present in plant-based foods; however, it is present in eggs and cheeses (especially Emmental, Edam and Cheddar), and, to a lesser extent, milk. Shellfish (such as clams, cockles, winkles, mussels, scallops and oysters) are a very rich source of vitamin B$^{12}$, as are fatty fish, such as sardines, kippers, salmon and tuna. Vitamin B$^{12}$ is also present in eggs.

## Folate
Folate is present in many green vegetables (for example, broccoli, Brussels sprouts, spinach and French beans) as well as wheat germ, nuts (especially peanuts, hazelnuts and walnuts), sesame seeds, fish, eggs and cheese.

## Vitamin C
Present in vegetables (peppers, kale, broccoli, Brussels sprouts, mangetout), and fruit (especially lemons, limes, oranges, blackcurrants and strawberries).

## Vitamin D
This vitamin is relatively unusual as the body can manufacture vitamin D from sunlight. The highest dietary sources are fatty

fish (herring, mackerel, sardines, tuna and salmon) and, to a lesser degree, cheese and eggs.

## Vitamin E
Once again, fatty fish are a good source of this essential vitamin, as well as wheat germ, shellfish, squid, vegetable oils and nuts.

## Vitamin K
Vitamin K is another vitamin which can be manufactured within the body, in this case by bacteria in the intestine. The richest dietary sources are found in green vegetables, especially broccoli, kale, Brussels sprouts, lettuce, cabbage and spinach.

# Minerals
Minerals are natural elements which are present in many foods. The following is not intended to be a comprehensive list of all of the minerals essential for health, but rather an indication of how easy it is to obtain essential minerals simply by following a diet low in refined carbohydrates but with virtually no restrictions on other foods.

| Calcium | Iodine | Potassium |
|---|---|---|
| Chromium | Iron | Sodium |
| Copper | Magnesium | Sulphur |

# Chapter 7  Foods included and foods excluded

Having explained the medical basis of the diet, it is relatively simple to summarise the foods which comprise the diet. As you will quickly realise, this diet is not simply based on excluding carbohydrates; on the contrary, many foods high in carb content (such as pasta and rice) are included in moderation by taking account of the Glycaemic Index and the subsequent effect on insulin production. Similarly, dairy products with a low carbohydrate content are restricted because of their potential to produce a higher insulin response (than their carb content would indicate) in some people.

In other words, this low-carb diet takes account of the many variable factors other than simply the carb content which make up a healthy weight-loss diet. Of course, you don't need to be concerned about these many variables; the diet is designed to ensure that, provided you adhere to its simple principles, you will be healthy and slim – without being hungry!

But, obviously, an inevitable consequence of including many foods of differing carb contents and Glycaemic Indices is that you must count the carb content for each day. Whichever foods you include in your diet, you must adhere to a maximum of 40–50 grams carbohydrate per day. The carbohydrate contents of all of the restricted foods are detailed in *The Ultimate Diet Counter* (published by Vermilion). All of the meals in this book (and our previous books) have the carb content of each meal carefully described.

So if you have a breakfast with a carb content of 25 grams, for example, or if you wish to enjoy a delicious low-carb dessert after dinner which may have a carb content of 20–30 grams, simply adjust your other meals for the day to take account of this and you will easily keep to the 50-gram carb daily limit. There are many meals with a very low carb content so it is really quite easy to keep to this diet. The following guidelines will ensure healthy dieting and successful weight loss.

## Low-carb foods included without restriction

- Poultry
- Fish
- Shellfish
- Most vegetables (except potatoes, parsnips and, to a lesser extent, carrots)
- Salads
- Herbs and spices
- Water/tea/low-calorie soft drinks
- Artificial sweeteners

## Low-carb foods included with some restriction

- Cheese – restrict to no more than 75 grams per day (0 carbs)
- Butter – 25 grams per day (0 carbs)
- Cream – 75 ml per day maximum
- Milk – 75 ml per day maximum
- Eggs – 1 egg per day
- Yoghurt – maximum 150 ml per day
- Oils – restrict to 'pure' oils such as extra-virgin olive oil or groundnut oils. Do not include corn oils or canola oils in the diet
- Mayonnaise – restrict to 2 tbsp per day
- Sauces
- Red wine/dry white wine – maximum 3 glasses per day

## Higher-carb foods included with significant restriction

- Wholemeal bread – 1 slice per day
- Wholemeal pasta – maintain restriction within daily total of 40–50 grams carb per day
- Arborio rice – maintain restriction within daily total of 40–50 grams carb per day
- Pulses
- Fruit
- Fruit juices
- Flour

## High-carb foods excluded from the diet

- All cakes, confectionery and biscuits
- Processed pies and pastries
- Breakfast cereals
- Beer/lager/cider/medium-sweet and sweet white wine/sherry/port

# Chapter **8** Healthy breakfast

The essence of successful dieting is *variety* in your diet. Most diets fail because of the monotonous repetition of meals which ultimately become unpalatable. In a low-GI/low-carb diet, this is impossible because there is such a diverse variety of meals available to suit every taste and lifestyle – no matter how hectic!

## Healthy low-GI/low-carb breakfast

All of the low-carb breakfast recipes included in our previous books are, by definition, low-GI. The purpose of this section is to discuss the wide range of healthy foods available in the low-GI/low-carb repertoire, and in particular to emphasise how easy it is to include healthy fruits and smoothies into the diet – provided you count the carb content.

## Refreshing juices

One of the many untrue criticisms of a low-carb diet is that it excludes fruit and vegetables and therefore must be unhealthy. In fact, there is absolutely no necessity to restrict most vegetables, and the restriction (not exclusion) of fruit does not affect the essential daily requirements for vitamins or minerals in any way whatsoever. This is most easily demonstrated by the inclusion of refreshing fruit and vegetable juices for breakfast.

It is important to dispel some of the (many) myths surrounding the place of fruit in a low-carb diet. First, it is *not* necessary to completely exclude fruit from a low-carb diet, merely to *restrict* fruit during the weight-loss phase. This means that you can enjoy fruit – or obviously fruit juices – provided you maintain your intake to less than 40 grams of carbohydrate per day.

The second myth is that you must consume large amounts of fruit juices for health. This is simply not correct. All of the vitamins and minerals present in fruit are also present in vegetables, and it is much more enjoyable (and refreshing) to add water to freshly squeezed juices. We have provided recipes for approximately 70 ml per person, which is about half the 'normal' amount of juice per portion. This may either be consumed undiluted, or diluted with cold spring water to taste. You can even double the amount of freshly squeezed juice if you wish; most recipes contain 8–12 grams per person and you can increase this, provided you keep to less than 40 grams of total carbohydrate per day.

### Raspberry and grapefruit
For 2     150 grams raspberries
          1 small grapefruit, segmented and deseeded

- *Juice the raspberries and grapefruit segments and serve immediately.*

*Carbohydrate content per serving: 9 grams*

### Melon and blueberries
For 2     ½ honeydew melon, peeled and segmented
          100 grams blueberries

- *Juice the melon and blueberries and serve immediately.*

*Carbohydrate content per serving: 11 grams*

**Watercress and carrot**

For 2   100 grams watercress
2 large carrots, peeled, topped and tailed and
   chopped
1 lemon quartered

• *Juice the ingredients and serve immediately.*

*Carbohydrate content per serving: **8** grams*

**Melon and lemon**

For 2   ½ honeydew melon, peeled and chopped
Juice of 1 freshly squeezed lemon
75 ml cold spring water

• *Juice the melon.*
• *Stir in the lemon juice and cold spring water, and
serve immediately.*

*Carbohydrate content per serving: **8** grams*

**Strawberry and pear**

For 2   100 grams strawberries
1 medium pear, stone removed and chopped

• *Juice the strawberries and pear segments and serve
immediately.*

*Carbohydrate content per serving: **11** grams*

### Avocado, tomato and basil

*For 2*  1 small Hass avocado, stone removed, peeled and chopped
3 medium plum tomatoes on-the-vine, chopped
6–8 large basil leaves, washed and finely chopped

- *Blend the ingredients and serve immediately.*

*Carbohydrate content per serving: **4** grams*

### Citrus and ginger

*For 2*  1 medium orange, peeled, segmented and deseeded
3 slices of fresh root ginger, peeled and chopped
1 tbsp freshly squeezed lime juice
15 grapes
75 ml cold spring water
Sprig of mint, to garnish

- *Juice the orange segments, ginger, lime juice and grapes.*
- *Stir in the cold spring water.*
- *Serve immediately, garnished with a sprig of mint.*

*Carbohydrate content per serving: **10** grams*

### Strawberry and blackberry

*For 2*  100 grams strawberries
100 grams blackberries

- *Juice the berries and serve immediately.*

*Carbohydrate content per serving: **9** grams*

## Melon and mint

For 2    1 medium, ripe Galia melon, peeled, deseeded
and chopped
3 tbsp freshly squeezed lemon juice
1 tbsp fresh mint leaves
Sprigs of fresh mint, to garnish

- *Put the melon, lemon juice and mint leaves into a blender, and purée.*
- *Serve immediately, garnished with fresh mint leaves.*

*Carbohydrate content per serving: **14** grams*

........................................................

## Carrot and apple

For 2    1 large carrot, peeled, topped and tailed and chopped
1 medium apple, cored and chopped
1 tsp orange zest

- *Juice the carrot, apple and orange zest and serve immediately.*

*Carbohydrate content per serving: **8** grams*

........................................................

## Peach and orange

For 2    1 medium peach, stone removed
1 medium orange, peeled, segmented and deseeded

- *Juice the peach and orange segments.*
- *Strain and serve immediately.*

*Carbohydrate content per serving: **9** grams*

## Kiwi and orange

For 2    2 kiwi fruit, peeled and chopped
1 orange, peeled and segmented
1 tsp orange zest
6 mint leaves
Sprig of mint, to garnish

- *Juice the ingredients.*
- *Stir and serve immediately, garnished with a sprig of mint.*

*Carbohydrate content per serving: **12** grams*

Of course, although the combination of various fruits and vegetable juices can be delicious, you can also enjoy pure juices of single fruits, either undiluted or with added spring water. Keep the carb count to less than 40 grams per day and the way you enjoy your (healthy) carbs is up to you!

A quick indicator of the carb content of various fruits is as follows:

## Carb grams

| | | | |
|---|---|---|---|
| Apple | 10 | Melon (100 grams) | |
| Apricot | 7 | Honeydew | 6 |
| Blackberries (100 grams) | 12 | Rock | 5 |
| Blueberries (100 grams) | 13 | Watermelon | 5 |
| Cherries (100 grams) | 12 | Nectarine | 7 |
| Gooseberries (100 grams) | 13 | Orange | 10 |
| Grapefruit (100 grams) | 10 | Passion fruit | 3 |
| Grapes (100 grams) | | Peach | 8 |
| Black grapes | 15 | Pear | 16 |
| Green grapes | 12 | Pineapple (100 grams) | 8 |
| Kiwi fruit | 7 | Plum | 8 |
| Lemon | 3 | Raspberries (100 grams) | 5 |
| Lime | 1 | Rhubarb (100 grams) | 1 |
| Mandarin | 4 | Satsuma | 7 |
| | | Strawberries (100 grams) | 6 |

# Smoothies

Yet another of the myths of the low-carb diet is that smoothies are excluded because of the sugar content of milk or yoghurt. Once again, this is nonsense! Milk (whether full fat, semi-skimmed or skimmed) contains approximately 5 grams of carbohydrate per 100 ml and natural yoghurt about 6 grams per 100 ml. Simple restriction of the amount of yoghurt or milk allows smoothies to be included in your low-carb diet easily.

**Mint and cucumber**

For 2   1 tbsp chopped mint leaves
1 medium English cucumber, peeled, deseeded and chopped
200 ml natural yoghurt

- *Blend together the mint, cucumber and yoghurt and serve immediately.*

*Carbohydrate content per serving: **12** grams*

**Raspberry and orange**

For 2   100 grams raspberries
100 ml natural yoghurt
100 ml freshly squeezed orange juice

- *Blend together the raspberries and yoghurt.*
- *Add the orange juice, blend until smooth and serve immediately.*

*Carbohydrate content per serving: **9** grams*

## Mango and lemon

For 2   150 ml milk, chilled
        1 medium fresh mango, peeled, stone removed and
           chopped
        2 tbsp freshly squeezed lemon juice
        2 tsp runny honey
        Fresh mint leaves, to garnish

- *Blend together the milk, mango, lemon juice and honey until smooth.*
- *Serve immediately, garnished with fresh mint leaves.*

*Carbohydrate content per serving:* **25** *grams*

• • • • • • • • • • • • • • • • • • • • • • • • • • • • • • • • • • • • • • • • • • • • • • • • • • • • • • • • • •

## Berry surprise

For 2   100 grams blackberries
        100 grams blueberries
        100 ml natural yoghurt, chilled
        Crushed ice

- *Blend together the blackberries, blueberries, yoghurt and ice, and serve immediately.*

*Carbohydrate content per serving:* **16** *grams*

## Citrus

For 2   3 tbsp freshly squeezed lemon juice
2 tbsp freshly squeezed lime juice
2 tsp caster sugar
150 ml natural yoghurt, chilled

- *Blend together the lemon juice, lime juice, caster sugar and yoghurt, and serve immediately.*

*Carbohydrate content per serving: **11** grams*

## Strawberry and whey

For 2   150 grams strawberries (or raspberries)
50 grams whey protein powder
100 ml water

- *Blend together the strawberries, whey protein and water, and serve immediately.*

*Carbohydrate content per serving: **12** grams*

# Porridge and yoghurt

Or course, when you *count* the carbs in a low-carb diet, rather than simply excluding any higher-carb foods, you can include porridge and yoghurt with fresh fruit for breakfast – simply make sure that you balance your daily carb content to be within the 50-gram limit.

**Porridge**

For 2    400 ml water, boiled
3 tbsp oatmeal
2 tsp granulated sugar (optional)
8 tbsp full-cream milk

- *Pour the water into a medium saucepan, bring to the boil and stir in the oatmeal.*
- *Simmer gently for 20–25 minutes.*
- *Mix in the sugar (optional) and milk and serve immediately.*

*Carbohydrate content per serving:* **25** *grams*
(**20** *grams without added sugar*)

**Fresh fruit with natural yoghurt**

For 2    1 medium apple, peeled, cored and chopped
1 medium orange, peeled, deseeded and chopped
100 grams fresh strawberries
100 ml natural yoghurt

- *Mix together the chopped apple, orange and strawberries in a medium bowl.*
- *Transfer to breakfast bowls, pour over the yoghurt and serve immediately.*

*Carbohydrate content per serving:* **19** *grams*

# Hot breakfast

A healthy and nutritious hot breakfast can easily be incorporated into the most hectic of lifestyles.

### Basil tomatoes with flaked smoked trout

For 2    2 beefsteak tomatoes (or 4 medium tomatoes), halved
1 tbsp chopped fresh basil
Balsamic vinegar, few drops
Extra-virgin olive oil, few drops
2 small smoked trout
Freshly ground black pepper

- *Top the tomato halves with chopped fresh basil.*
- *Drizzle the balsamic vinegar and extra-virgin olive oil over the tomatoes, and place on a grill tray.*
- *Grill under a hot grill (no closer than 8–10 cm from the grill) for 4–5 minutes.*

*At the same time*

- *Place the smoked trout in a microwave-safe dish and microwave on 'high' for 2 minutes, or place in an oven-safe dish, cover with pierced aluminium foil and cook in the centre of a preheated oven at 180°C (gas mark 4) for 10–12 minutes.*

- *Flake the smoked trout and serve with the grilled basil tomatoes.*
- *Season to taste with freshly ground black pepper.*

*Carbohydrate content per serving:* **4** *grams*

## Chestnut mushrooms with herb butter

Chestnut mushrooms can be substituted with large flat mushrooms, or you can use 100 grams small brown (or button) mushrooms instead.

For 2
3 tbsp extra-virgin olive oil
4 large chestnut mushrooms, wiped and stalks removed
4 spring onions, chopped on the diagonal into 4–5 cm lengths
50 grams unsalted butter
1 tbsp chopped fresh basil leaves
Freshly ground black pepper

* *Heat the extra-virgin olive oil in a medium frying pan and gently sauté the mushrooms and spring onions for 3–4 minutes, turning once.*

*At the same time*
* *Melt the butter in a small saucepan, then stir in the basil.*
* *Heat through gently for 1–2 minutes.*

* *Serve the mushrooms and spring onions onto warm plates, spoon over the herb butter and season to taste.*

*Carbohydrate content per serving: **6** grams*

## Eggs Florentine

For 2    75 grams unsalted butter
500 grams fresh spinach leaves, rinsed, drained and stalks removed
2 tbsp chopped fresh basil leaves
4 large, fresh free-range eggs
2 tbsp Parmesan cheese, grated
Freshly ground black pepper

- *Melt the butter in a large saucepan, then gently sauté the spinach and basil, over a low heat, for 1–2 minutes until just softened. Not too long, or it will disappear!*
- *Transfer the spinach mixture to a shallow, oven-safe dish and smooth evenly over the base.*
- *Form four hollow shapes in the spinach.*
- *Break an egg into the centre of each hollow.*
- *Sprinkle ½ tbsp of Parmesan cheese over each egg, season to taste with black pepper and cook in the centre of a preheated oven at 180°C (gas mark 4) for 12–15 minutes, depending on the oven.*
- *Serve immediately.*

*Carbohydrate content per serving:* **6** *grams*

**Char-grilled mushrooms with scrambled eggs**

For 2     1 tbsp unsalted butter
           1 tbsp Dijon mustard
           2 large flat mushrooms
           2 large free-range eggs
           1 tbsp freshly chopped chives
           Freshly ground black pepper

- *Melt the butter in a small saucepan and mix in the Dijon mustard.*
- *Spread the mixture over the mushrooms and grill under a hot grill (no closer than 8–10 cm from the grill) for about 5 minutes.*

*At the same time*
- *Prepare the scrambled eggs.*

- *Place a mushroom in the centre of each plate and top with scrambled eggs.*
- *Garnish with chopped chives and season to taste.*

*Carbohydrate content per serving: **3** grams*

## Kippers with tomatoes

For 2      3 tbsp extra-virgin olive oil
2 medium kippers
4 medium plum tomatoes, halved
Freshly ground black pepper

- *Heat the extra-virgin olive oil in a medium frying pan and add the kippers and tomatoes.*
- *Cook the kippers and tomatoes for 4–5 minutes, turning once.*
- *Season to taste and serve immediately.*

*Carbohydrate content per serving:* **5** *grams*

**Grilled apples with pineapple and mint**

For 2    2 large Royal Gala apples (or similar, to taste)
25 grams unsalted butter
Pinch of cinnamon
100 grams fresh pineapple, chopped
1 tbsp chopped fresh mint leaves

- *Peel and core the apples, then slice finely, place on a grill tray and dot with butter.*
- *Grill under a medium grill (no closer than 8–10 cm from the grill) for 2–3 minutes, turning once.*
- *Sprinkle over a little cinnamon, spoon the chopped pineapple onto the apples and garnish with fresh mint. Serve immediately.*

*Carbohydrate content per serving: **18** grams*

In this context, we have published a series of books which are complementary to the present book. There are many standard breakfasts that have been described previously and which we have no intention of repeating here, but you should be aware of the sources of these recipes in order to expand your repertoire (and variety) of meals. Typical recipes (which can obviously be used in combination with any other low-carb ingredient) previously described include:

**The New High Protein Diet**
- Scrambled eggs (with multiple fillings)
- Boiled eggs
- Omelette (with multiple fillings)
- Poached eggs
- Eggs Benedict
- Fried eggs
- Lemon sole
- Baked haddock (with Swiss cheese)
- Kippers
- Mushrooms on toast
- Toasted cheese
- Continental breakfast

**The New High Protein Diet Cookbook**
- Savoury crêpes
- Haddock and Parmesan
- Mushroom and chicken
- Breakfast tortilla
- Bagel delights
- Sun-dried tomatoes and herbs
- Spinach and mackerel
- Breakfast drinks

- Citrus stinger
- Watermelon delight
- Apple and strawberry appetiser
- Citrus carrot
- Raspberry and apple energiser
- Berry zest
- Kiwi surprise
- Tomato juice
- Mango and strawberry milkshake
- Blueberry milkshake

**The New High Protein Healthy Fast Food Diet**
Healthy diet solutions for busy people on-the-run including take-away and bistro breakfasts.

# Chapter **9** Mid-day revival

Lunch can be the most difficult meal of the day on a low-carb/low-GI diet because it is so dependent on circumstances which you may be unable to predict. Obviously, if you are able to be at home then it is much easier to keep low-carb, but this is an advantage denied to many of us. If you understand the low-carb options available in every situation – no matter how hectic your lifestyle – you will find that maintaining your diet is so much easier. When the recipes in this book are combined with the others from our complementary books, you can see that this is quite simply the most varied and delicious diet ever devised – apart from being the healthiest! With diverse recipes including fish, shellfish, poultry, crêpes, soufflés and soups – and including many potential variations with Chinese, Indian, Thai and Mexican foods – and the healthy 'fast-food' options of deli salad lunch-boxes and open sandwiches, there really is the opportunity for everyone to enjoy this healthy diet.

## Soups

For many of us, the preparation of home-made soups is not an option because of time constraints. In actual fact, home-made soup can be prepared quite simply and can be frozen for later use, thereby providing a nutritious and healthy low-GI/low-carb option for several later meals. This is why we have included a delicious range of easy-to-prepare, nutritious home-made soups.

**Tomato and aubergine soup**

For 2   1 large aubergine
2 tbsp extra-virgin olive oil
1 medium red onion, peeled and diced
1 medium garlic clove, peeled and finely chopped
2 medium tomatoes on-the-vine, peeled, deseeded
   and finely chopped
1 tsp tomato purée
1 slice of fresh ginger root, peeled and finely chopped
400 ml vegetable stock
1 tbsp chopped fresh coriander leaves
1 tbsp freshly squeezed lemon juice
2 tbsp single cream
Pinch of sea salt
Freshly ground black pepper

- *Brush the aubergine with some of the extra-virgin olive oil, prick the skin, then place on an oven tray and cook in the centre of a preheated oven at 200°C (gas mark 6) for about 20 minutes.*

*At the same time*
- *Heat the remaining extra-virgin olive oil in a large saucepan and sauté the onion and garlic for 3–4 minutes.*
- *Stir in the tomatoes, tomato purée, ginger root, stock, coriander and lemon juice, and simmer gently for 5 minutes.*

- *Remove the aubergine from the oven and allow to cool for 5 minutes.*
- *Chop the aubergine into quarters and scoop out the contents, which should then be added to the soup.*

- *Purée the soup.*
- *Stir in the cream, return the soup to the saucepan, season to taste and heat through gently (do not boil), then serve immediately.*

*Carbohydrate content per serving: **10** grams*

**Hearty pumpkin and tomato soup**

For 2    2 tbsp extra-virgin olive oil
         3 shallots, peeled and chopped
         200 grams of butternut pumpkin, peeled, deseeded
             and chopped into 2–3 cm cubes
         2 large plum tomatoes on-the-vine, peeled, deseeded
             and chopped
         2 slices of fresh ginger root, peeled and finely chopped
         400 ml vegetable stock
         1 tbsp chopped fresh basil
         1 tbsp chopped fresh flat-leaf parsley
         Pinch of sea salt
         Freshly ground black pepper

- *Heat the extra-virgin olive oil in a large saucepan and sauté the shallots for 2–3 minutes.*
- *Add the pumpkin and cook over a medium heat for 5–7 minutes, stirring frequently.*
- *Stir in the tomatoes, ginger, stock, basil and parsley, season to taste and simmer for 30–35 minutes.*
- *Serve immediately.*

*Carbohydrate content per serving: **12 grams***

**Creamy mushroom soup**

For 2   1 tbsp extra-virgin olive oil
2 shallots, peeled and finely chopped
1 garlic clove, peeled and finely chopped
60 grams button mushrooms, wiped and finely sliced
½ tbsp plain flour
150 ml chicken (or vegetable) stock
150 ml full-cream milk
Pinch of salt
Freshly ground black pepper
1 tbsp medium sherry (or Marsala)
1 tbsp freshly chopped flat-leaf parsley, to garnish

- *Heat the extra-virgin olive oil in a medium saucepan and gently sauté the shallots and garlic for 2–3 minutes.*
- *Stir in the mushrooms and cook for a further 2–3 minutes.*
- *Remove from the heat and stir in the flour.*
- *Return to a gentle heat and stir in the stock and milk.*
- *Season to taste then simmer gently for 2–3 minutes, but do not allow to boil.*
- *Purée the soup.*
- *Stir in the medium sherry (or Marsala) and serve immediately, garnished with freshly chopped flat-leaf parsley.*

*Carbohydrate content per serving: **12** grams*

**Spicy tomato and lentil soup**

For 2   100 grams dried red lentils
2 tbsp extra-virgin olive oil
1 medium red onion, peeled and chopped
1 garlic clove, peeled and chopped
½ tsp ground cumin
½ tsp garam masala
½ tsp ground coriander
Pinch of cayenne pepper
500 ml organic vegetable stock
2 tbsp tomato purée
6 Dutch campari tomatoes, peeled and halved
Pinch of rock salt
Freshly ground black pepper
1 tbsp chopped fresh coriander leaves

- *Place the lentils in a medium bowl, cover with cold water and soak overnight, then drain the lentils before use.*
- *Heat the extra-virgin olive oil in a large saucepan and sauté the onion and garlic for 2 minutes.*
- *Stir in the cumin, garam masala, coriander, pepper and lentils, and cook for 2–3 minutes.*
- *Stir in the vegetable stock, tomato purée and tomatoes, season to taste and simmer gently for 35–40 minutes.*
- *Stir in the fresh coriander leaves and heat through gently for a further 5 minutes, then serve immediately.*

*Carbohydrate content per serving: **19** grams*

**Seafood and herb chowder**

This is more of a meal than a soup and can include a variety of
different fish and shellfish: haddock, cod, bream, sole, scallops,
clams, mussels, prawns or calamari are just a few of the almost
unrestricted possibilities in this meal.

For 2
1 kg mixed fish and shellfish
1 tbsp chopped fresh coriander leaves
1 tbsp chopped fresh flat-leaf parsley
1 tbsp chopped fresh chives
8 black peppercorns
250 ml fish stock
200 ml dry white wine
1 tbsp extra-virgin olive oil
2 shallots, peeled and chopped
1 large garlic clove, peeled and chopped
2 slices of fresh ginger root, peeled and chopped
200 grams tinned plum tomatoes
Freshly ground black pepper

- *Chop the fish into 3–5 cm chunks and place in a
  large casserole dish.*
- *Scrub the shellfish, discarding any open shells, and
  add to the casserole dish.*
- *Add the coriander, parsley, chives and peppercorns
  and stir in the stock and wine.*
- *Cover and cook in the centre of a pre-heated oven at
  180°C (gas mark 4) for 15 minutes.*
- *Discard any unopened shellfish.*

*Just before the seafood is ready*
- *Heat the extra-virgin olive oil in a large, deep frying
  pan and sauté the shallots and garlic.*

- *Stir in the ginger and tomatoes, then add the cooked seafood and its stock.*
- *Season to taste, simmer for 3–4 minutes, then serve immediately.*

*Carbohydrate content per serving: **8** grams*

**Hot and spicy tomato soup**

For 2    2 tbsp extra-virgin olive oil
1 medium red onion, peeled and diced
1 medium garlic clove, peeled and chopped
400 grams tinned peeled Roma tomatoes
1 tsp dried oregano
2 slices fresh ginger root, peeled and chopped
150 ml vegetable stock
1 tsp brown sugar
3–4 drops Tabasco sauce (optional)
1 tbsp chopped fresh basil
1 tbsp freshly squeezed lemon juice
Pinch of sea salt
Freshly ground black pepper
Small fresh basil leaves, to garnish

- *Heat the extra-virgin olive oil in a medium saucepan and sauté the onion and garlic for 2–3 minutes.*
- *Stir in the tomatoes, oregano and ginger, and simmer gently for 3–4 minutes.*
- *Add the stock, sugar, Tabasco sauce, basil and lemon juice, season to taste, and simmer for about 20 minutes.*
- *Purée the soup, then return to the saucepan and heat through gently.*
- *Serve immediately, garnished with fresh basil leaves.*

*Carbohydrate content per serving: **14** grams*

## Mascarpone and spinach soup

For 2    1 tbsp extra-virgin olive oil
2 shallots, peeled and chopped
1 medium garlic clove, peeled and chopped
200 grams fresh spinach leaves, washed
2 tbsp chopped fresh basil leaves
400 ml vegetable stock (such as Marigold Swiss
  vegetable bouillon powder)
100 grams Mascarpone cheese
Pinch of rock salt
Freshly ground black pepper
Fresh single cream (optional)

- *Heat the extra-virgin olive oil in a large saucepan and sauté the shallots and garlic for 2–3 minutes.*
- *Stir in the spinach, basil and the vegetable stock, and simmer gently for 20 minutes.*
- *Transfer to a blender and purée.*
- *Return the purée to a clean saucepan, stir in the Mascarpone cheese and simmer gently, stirring frequently, until the cheese has melted.*
- *Season to taste and serve immediately with a swirl of fresh cream (optional).*

*Carbohydrate content per serving: **10** grams*

**Mulligatawny soup**

For 2    2 tbsp extra-virgin olive oil
1 small brown onion, peeled and diced
1 garlic clove, peeled and grated
2 slices of fresh root ginger, peeled and finely
    chopped
¼ tsp chilli powder (optional)
½ tsp ground cumin
½ tsp ground turmeric
½ tsp ground fenugreek
250 ml vegetable stock
1 tsp freshly squeezed lime juice
1 tbsp chopped fresh coriander leaves
Pinch of sea salt
Freshly ground black pepper
70 ml coconut milk

- *Heat the extra-virgin olive oil in a medium saucepan and sauté the onion and garlic for 2–3 minutes.*
- *Add the ginger, chilli, cumin, turmeric and fenugreek, and stir-fry for 2 minutes.*
- *Stir in the vegetable stock, lime juice and coriander, season to taste and simmer gently for 5–7 minutes.*
- *Stir in the coconut milk and heat through gently.*
- *Serve immediately.*

*Carbohydrate content per serving: **7** grams*

### Chilled cucumber soup

For 2　　1 large cucumber, peeled and diced
400 ml vegetable stock
1½ tbsp chopped fresh chives
Pinch of sea salt
Freshly ground black pepper
100 ml single cream

- *Add the cucumber to the stock in a large saucepan, bring to the boil, then reduce the heat and simmer gently for 30 minutes.*
- *Stir in a tbsp of chopped fresh chives, season to taste and purée.*
- *Return the puréed soup to the pan, stir in the cream and heat through gently for about 4–5 minutes.*
- *Chill in the fridge for 2 hours then serve, garnished with the remaining chopped chives.*

*Carbohydrate content per serving:* **16** *grams*

**Oriental soup**

For 2     450 ml chicken stock
2 slices fresh ginger root, peeled and grated
100 grams tofu, chopped into 2 cm cubes
50 grams cooked prawns, shelled
50 grams bamboo shoots, drained and finely sliced
2 spring onions, chopped into 1–2 cm lengths on the
diagonal
Pinch of sea salt
Freshly ground black pepper
2 cooked tiger prawns

- *Bring the chicken stock to the boil, then add the ginger, tofu, prawns, bamboo shoots and spring onions.*
- *Season to taste and simmer gently for 15 minutes.*
- *Serve immediately, garnished with cooked tiger prawns.*

*Carbohydrate content per serving: **8** grams*

## Tofu and red pepper soup

For 2    450 ml vegetable stock
         2 slices fresh ginger root, peeled and grated
         100 grams tofu, chopped into 2 cm cubes
         1 small red pepper, deseeded and finely sliced
         50 grams bamboo shoots, drained and finely sliced
         2 spring onions, chopped into 1–2 cm lengths on the
             diagonal
         Pinch of sea salt
         Freshly ground black pepper
         ½ tbsp freshly chopped coriander leaves

- *Bring the vegetable stock to the boil, then add the ginger, tofu, red pepper, bamboo shoots and spring onions.*
- *Season to taste and simmer gently for 15 minutes.*
- *Serve immediately and sprinkle over freshly chopped coriander leaves.*

*Carbohydrate content per serving: **11** grams*

Other soup recipes included in previous books include:

**The New High Protein Diet**
- Avocado
- Hot pepper and coriander
- Carrot and coriander
- Cream of chicken
- Carrot and orange
- Gazpacho

**The New High Protein Diet Cookbook**
- Borscht
- Pumpkin and coriander
- Chilled leek and potato
- Creamy Gruyère
- Lemon and chicken
- Creamy spinach and coriander
- Broccoli and basil
- French onion
- Watercress

# Light lunch

### Pickled herrings with beetroot

For 2
2 spring onions, finely diced
½ Lebanese cucumber, diced
1 tbsp freshly squeezed lemon juice
2 pickled herrings (roll mops), drained and sliced into thin strips
100 ml crème fraîche (or soured cream)
Freshly ground black pepper
1 tbsp chopped fresh chives
100 grams pickled beetroot

- *Mix together the spring onions, cucumber, lemon juice and sliced herrings in a medium bowl.*
- *Stir in the crème fraîche.*
- *Spoon onto plates, season to taste and garnish with chopped chives.*
- *Serve immediately with pickled beetroot.*

*Carbohydrate content per serving: **10** grams*

**Toasted sesame seeds with avocado aioli**

For 2    1 large, ripe Hass avocado, halved lengthways and
          stone removed
          60 ml aioli
          1 tbsp freshly squeezed lemon juice
          75 grams small broccoli florets
          1 tbsp sesame seeds
          1 tbsp freshly chopped chives
          Freshly ground black pepper

- *Scoop out the avocado and mix with 60 ml aioli and lemon juice.*

*At the same time*
- *Lightly steam the broccoli florets for 3–4 minutes (or microwave for 2–3 minutes on 'high').*

*And*
- *Toast (dry-fry) the sesame seeds in a small frying pan for 1 minute.*

- *Combine the avocado and aioli with the broccoli florets and spoon into small bowls.*
- *Top with the toasted sesame seeds and chopped chives, and season to taste.*
- *Serve immediately.*

*Carbohydrate content per serving: **5** grams*

**Cod roe with cucumber**

For 2    75 grams Philadelphia cheese
50 ml crème fraîche
Freshly ground black pepper
½ medium cucumber, sliced into ½ cm rounds
30 grams cod roe
100 grams rocket and watercress salad

- *Mix together the Philadelphia cheese and crème fraîche in a medium bowl and season to taste.*
- *Lay the cucumber slices individually on a plate.*
- *Spoon a little of the mixture in the centre of each cucumber slice.*
- *Top with a little cod roe (not too much; this has a very 'rich' flavour).*
- *Serve with rocket and watercress salad.*

*Carbohydrate content per serving:* **14** *grams*

**Angel hair pasta with Italian sauce**

For 2    1 tbsp extra-virgin olive oil
1 medium shallot, peeled and finely chopped
1 garlic clove, peeled and finely chopped
2 slices fresh ginger root, peeled and finely chopped
50 grams button mushrooms, wiped and sliced
100 ml dry white wine
1 tbsp freshly squeezed lime juice
1 tsp tomato purée
1 tsp dried oregano
60 grams angel hair pasta
1 tbsp chopped fresh flat-leaf parsley
Freshly ground black pepper

- *Heat the extra-virgin olive oil in a medium frying pan and sauté the shallot, garlic, ginger and mushrooms for 2 minutes.*
- *Add the dry white wine, lime juice, tomato purée and oregano, and simmer gently for 2–3 minutes.*

*At the same time*
- *Cook the angel hair pasta in a large pan of boiling water for 2 minutes.*

- *Toss the pasta with the sauce, stir in the parsley and season to taste.*

*Carbohydrate content per serving: **27 grams***

**Tangy baked kippers**

This delicious meal could not be any quicker, simpler – or healthier. With essential amino acids, omega-3 fatty acids, calcium and vitamin D from kippers complemented by the vitamin C from citrus fruits, this is nutritionally perfect.

For 2     1 tbsp extra-virgin olive oil
4 tbsp freshly squeezed lemon juice
1 bay leaf
Freshly ground black pepper
2 medium kippers, heads and tails removed
100 grams baby spinach leaves
50 grams pine nuts

- *Add the extra-virgin olive oil, lemon juice, bay leaf and pepper to a screw-top jar and mix thoroughly.*
- *Place the kipper fillets, skin-side down, in a single layer in a shallow dish.*
- *Marinate in the fridge for 3–4 hours.*
- *Cover the dish with pierced aluminium foil and cook in the centre of a pre-heated oven at 180°C (Gas 4) for 15–20 minutes.*
- *Serve with a salad of baby spinach leaves and garnish with pine nuts.*

*Carbohydrate content per serving: **4** grams*

## Seared scallops with watercress salad

For 2     2 tbsp extra-virgin olive oil
8 medium fresh scallops, corals removed
50 grams watercress
50 grams rocket
Balsamic vinaigrette (page 222)
Freshly ground black pepper
1 tbsp chopped fresh chives

- *Heat the extra-virgin olive oil in a medium frying pan and cook the scallops for 4 minutes, turning once.*
- *Lay the scallops on a bed of mixed watercress and rocket leaves, and drizzle over a little Balsamic vinaigrette.*
- *Season to taste with freshly ground black pepper, garnish with chopped chives and serve immediately.*

*Carbohydrate content per serving: **5** grams*

**Penne rigate with mixed veggies**

For 2    25 grams mangetout
25 grams broccoli florets
1 small red pepper, deseeded and finely sliced
40 grams wholemeal penne rigate
75 ml double cream
1 tbsp freshly chopped basil
1 tbsp freshly grated Parmesan cheese
Freshly ground black pepper

- *Lightly steam the mangetout, broccoli florets and red pepper for 4–5 minutes (or microwave on 'high' for 2–3 minutes).*

*At the same time*

- *Cook the penne rigate (page 126).*
- *Mix together the double cream and basil.*

- *Stir in the mangetout, broccoli and red pepper into the penne rigate, stir in the cream and Parmesan cheese, and season to taste with freshly ground black pepper.*

*Carbohydrate content per serving: **20** grams*

**Sesame tiger prawns with Chinese leaves**

For 2 
1 tbsp sesame seeds
1 tbsp sesame oil
8 raw tiger prawns, peeled and deveined
1 green chilli, deseeded and finely chopped (optional)
3 slices fresh root ginger, peeled and finely chopped
2 tbsp rice wine or dry sherry (optional)
6 Chinese leaves
Pinch of sea salt
Freshly ground black pepper

- *Dry stir-fry the sesame seeds, then set aside.*
- *Heat the sesame oil in a wok and stir-fry the prawns, chilli, ginger and rice wine or sherry for 3–4 minutes.*

*At the same time*
- *Lightly steam the Chinese leaves for 3–4 minutes (or microwave on 'high' for 2–3 minutes).*

- *Serve the prawns on a bed of Chinese leaves, season to taste and drizzle over a few drops of sesame oil.*

*Carbohydrate content per serving: **4** grams*

We have described many other healthy low-GI/low-carb recipes which are ideally suited to this diet in previous books. In a book of this nature, which is attempting to bring together all of the multitude of varied healthy low-GI/low-carb recipes, it is essential to cross-reference to provide the variety without repetition. Of course, our previous low-carb books also contained recipes including beef, pork and lamb, but the recipes most appropriate to a red meat-free diet are the following:

## The New High Protein Diet

### Fish and shellfish

- Grilled/poached salmon with various sauces and salads
- Smoked salmon and sour cream salsa
- Salmon pâté
- Trout with lemon and pine nuts
- Trout teriyaki
- Baked trout with ginger and lime
- Trout with lemon Hollandaise sauce
- Lemon sole with pak choi
- Dover sole with herb sauce
- Tuna with herbs
- Tuna in dill mayonnaise with mangetout
- Tuna burrito
- Cod with basil and chives
- Cod with tomato and coriander salsa
- Cod with parsley sauce
- Swordfish steaks with lemon and garlic
- Smoked mackerel pâté
- Grilled mackerel with lime
- Mackerel with lemon and coriander
- Smoked mackerel with crushed black pepper
- Whiting with ginger and lime
- Soused herrings with radish and basil salad

- Haddock with peppers and ginger
- Poached haddock with mushroom and sherry sauce
- Prawns in garlic butter
- Tiger prawn salad with avocado lime dressing
- Tiger prawns with basil and tomatoes
- Prawns and avocado
- Hot and spicy prawns
- Prawns with rocket salad
- Chilli tiger prawns with mangetout
- Scallops with lime and ginger
- Scallops and asparagus with sweet chilli sauce
- Ginger scallops with mangetout
- Mussels in tomato sauce with oregano
- Mussels in garlic sauce

**Poultry**
- Tandoori-style chicken
- Ginger chicken with orange
- Chicken tikka
- Lemon chicken with cashew nuts
- Chicken with prosciutto
- Chicken korma
- Spicy chicken drumsticks
- Chicken with tomato and basil sauce
- Chicken burritos
- Tarragon chicken with tomato and avocado
- Roast duck with juniper berries and orange liqueur sauce

**The New High Protein Diet Cookbook**
**Fish/shellfish**
- Crab soufflé
- Creamy prawns with basil
- Salmon steaks with leek and lemon butter sauce
- Smoked haddock soufflé

- Scallop and calamari salad
- Smoked trout frittata
- Tuna with creamy herb sauce
- Egg mayonnaise with smoked salmon
- Shellfish with bok choy
- Salmon with watercress and mint sauce
- Crab and herb salad
- Baked trout with pine nut and almond butter
- Tiger prawns with coconut milk
- Parmesan salmon

**Poultry**

- Barbecue turkey salad
- Mozzarella chicken
- Basil pesto turkey with char-grilled vegetables and sesame seeds
- Barbecued turkey keftas with cucumber raita
- Chilli mayonnaise turkey with mangetout
- Turkey and avocado

### The New High Protein Healthy Fast Food Diet

For lunch-on-the-run there is an immense variety of potential options available – without resorting to the ubiquitous carbohydrate-based sandwiches, pittas, wraps, rice- and pasta-based meals, pizzas, burgers and fries. Healthy low-carb recipes and options for those with a hectic, busy lifestyle are described in detail in *The New High Protein Healthy Fast Food Diet*; here are some suggestions.

Probably the simplest solution for lunch-on-the-run is either a salad lunchbox or an open sandwich on a single slice of wholegrain bread, although alternatives include prawn mayonnaise, cooked chicken (legs, thighs, wings or breast), tuna with sweetcorn, coronation chicken, cheeses, smoked salmon and egg mayonnaise. All of the above are available pre-packaged in the delicatessen section of many supermarkets, which even provide disposable cutlery.

A salad lunchbox can either be prepared at home or purchased at the local deli. The quantity of these foods is virtually unrestricted, so enjoy as much salad and fillings as you like. Always remember to add vinaigrette, dressing (low-carb, naturally) or mayonnaise to your salad, as this not only provides essential fats in your diet but also slows the absorption of the food, reducing insulin release and staving off hunger for hours! All salad foods are included, with just a slight restriction on tomatoes (one medium or four cherry tomatoes per meal). The *New High Protein Healthy Fast Food Diet* obviously includes many additional recipes with beef, pork, ham and lamb.

The same fillings are equally applicable to both lunchboxes or open sandwiches. Here are some suggestions – but the potential variations are virtually unlimited. In each case this will be either on a bed of mixed salad in a lunch box, or with a little salad in a sandwich.

- Chicken breast with chilli sauce
- Egg mayonnaise with fresh basil and chives
- Roast ham with Leerdammer cheese
- Avocado with Bocconcini
- Tuna mayonnaise with basil and coriander
- Salmon with crème fraîche
- Greek salad
- Port Salut, courgettes and chives salad
- Tiger prawns with chilli and coriander vinaigrette
- Red pepper and sun-dried tomato salad
- Prawn mayonnaise
- Chicken tikka
- Guacamole
- Coronation chicken
- Avocado with tomato and mayonnaise
- Egg and cress
- Turkey breast with cranberry sauce

# Chapter 10 Evening posh nosh

The evening meal can be the easiest to incorporate into the low-GI lifestyle, as there is usually a little more time available to prepare this meal than either breakfast or lunch. Here is a selection of healthy – and delicious – low-GI/low-carb meals, most of which require a reasonably short preparation time. Of course, many of the recipes in Chapter 11 for vegetarians are equally suitable for everyone. An extensive list of alternative meat-free recipes included in the other books in the series is described at the end of Chapter 11.

## Avocado and smoked salmon with dill mayonnaise
Quick and simple – but highly nutritious and delicious!

For 2    Medium Hass avocado, peeled, stone removed and
             sliced
         75 grams smoked salmon, sliced into thin strips
         1 tbsp freshly squeezed lime juice
         Freshly ground black pepper

### Dill mayonnaise
         2 tbsp mayonnaise – commercial or home-made
         ½ tbsp finely chopped fresh dill

- *Divide avocado slices evenly between two plates and place in the centre.*
- *Lay several strips of smoked salmon on the avocado.*
- *Drizzle the lime juice over the salmon.*

*At the same time*
- *Mix together the mayonnaise and dill.*

- *Spoon the dill mayonnaise onto the salmon and season to taste with freshly ground black pepper.*

*Carbohydrate content per serving: **3** grams*

**Stir-fried tofu with mushrooms**

For 2

150 grams tofu, chopped into 2 cm cubes
3 tbsp extra-virgin olive oil
75 grams mangetout
75 grams bamboo shoots, sliced into thin strips
75 grams button mushrooms, wiped and halved
2 slices fresh ginger root, peeled and finely chopped
1 tbsp sesame seeds
Freshly ground black pepper

Marinade

1 tsp granulated sugar
3 tbsp light soy sauce
3 tbsp dry sherry

- *Make the marinade by mixing the ingredients together.*
- *Rinse the chopped tofu and pat dry, put it in the marinade and leave for 6–8 hours.*
- *Heat 2 tbsp extra-virgin olive oil in a wok and stir-fry the tofu and marinade for 2–3 minutes, then remove from the wok with a perforated spoon and set aside.*
- *Heat the remaining olive oil in the wok and stir-fry the mangetout, bamboo shoots, mushrooms and ginger for 2–3 minutes, then add the tofu and stir-fry for a final 2 minutes.*
- *Dry stir-fry the sesame seeds in a small saucepan for 1 minute.*
- *Season the tofu mixture to taste and serve immediately, garnished with the toasted sesame seeds.*

*Carbohydrate content per serving: **14** grams*

## Smoked salmon with fennel and dill

For 2
100 grams smoked salmon, finely sliced
1 tbsp freshly squeezed lime juice
1 tbsp Parmesan shavings
Freshly ground black pepper

### Cream sauce

75 ml fresh single cream
½ tbsp finely chopped fresh fennel
½ tbsp finely chopped fresh dill

- *Place the smoked salmon strips in the centre of the plates.*
- *Drizzle over a little lime juice.*
- *Mix together the cream, fennel and dill, and pour over the smoked salmon.*
- *Top with Parmesan shavings and season to taste with freshly ground black pepper.*

*Carbohydrate content per serving: **3** grams*

**Baked turkey with peppers and herbs**

For 2    1 small red pepper, deseeded and finely chopped
1 small yellow pepper, deseeded and finely chopped
1 tbsp chopped fresh basil
1 shallot, peeled and finely chopped
1 garlic clove, peeled and finely chopped
2 tbsp extra-virgin olive oil
250 grams sliced uncooked turkey breast
Freshly ground black pepper
100 grams mangetout

- *Mix together the chopped peppers, basil, shallot, garlic and olive oil in a medium bowl.*
- *Place the slices of turkey breast in an oven-safe dish and coat with the pepper mixture.*
- *Cover with pierced aluminium foil and cook in the centre of a preheated oven at 180°C (gas mark 4) for 30–35 minutes.*

*Just before the turkey is ready*
- *Lightly steam the mangetout for 4–5 minutes (or microwave on 'high' for 2–3 minutes).*
- *Season to taste and serve the turkey with the mangetout.*

*Carbohydrate content per serving: **8** grams*

## Pan-fried cod with herb butter

For 2
2 tbsp extra-virgin olive oil
2 cod fillets, approximately 150 grams each
75 grams unsalted butter
1 tbsp freshly chopped sage
1 tbsp freshly chopped dill
1 tbsp capers, drained and rinsed
75 grams fresh watercress
Freshly ground black pepper

- *Heat the extra-virgin olive oil in a medium frying pan and fry the cod for 4–5 minutes, turning once.*

*At the same time*
- *Melt the butter in a medium saucepan, stir in the sage, dill and capers, and heat gently for 2 minutes.*

- *Serve the cod with fresh watercress, drizzle the herb butter sauce over the fish, and season to taste.*

*Carbohydrate content per serving:* **4 grams**

**Coconut okra curry**

For 2    2 tbsp extra-virgin olive oil
150 grams okra, topped and tailed and halved
    lengthways
½ tsp ground coriander
½ tsp ground turmeric
½ tsp ground cumin
1 small red chilli, deseeded and finely chopped
    (optional)
3 slices of fresh ginger root, peeled and finely chopped
50 ml vegetable stock
200 ml natural yoghurt
50 ml coconut milk
1 tbsp freshly chopped coriander leaves
Freshly ground black pepper
Fresh coriander leaves, to garnish

- *Heat the extra-virgin olive oil in a medium frying pan and stir-fry the okra over a medium heat for 4–5 minutes.*
- *Stir in the ground coriander, turmeric, cumin, chilli and ginger and stir-fry for a further minute.*
- *Add the vegetable stock and simmer gently for 8–10 minutes.*
- *Stir in the yoghurt, coconut milk and fresh coriander, season to taste and heat through gently for about 2 minutes. Do not allow to boil.*
- *Serve immediately, garnished with fresh coriander leaves.*

*Carbohydrate content per serving: **9** grams*

**Griddled duck with lentil purée**

For 2    1 tbsp lentils
2 duck breast fillets, skin removed
2 tbsp extra-virgin olive oil
1 small red onion, peeled and diced
1 garlic clove, peeled and chopped
3 tbsp Madeira wine (or medium sherry)
2 tbsp chicken stock
200 gram tin of cooked chickpeas, drained
1 tbsp chopped fresh basil leaves
Freshly ground black pepper
1 tbsp chopped fresh chives

- *Place the lentils in a small bowl, cover with water and soak overnight, then drain.*
- *Add the lentils to a small saucepan, cover with cold water, bring to the boil and simmer for 30 minutes.*
- *Drain and set aside.*

*At the same time*

- *Slash each duck breast diagonally twice, then cook them on a griddle pan for 6–8 minutes (according to taste), turning once.*
- *Allow the duck fat to drain, then remove from the heat and set aside.*
- *Slice thinly when cool.*

*And*

- *Heat the extra-virgin olive oil in a medium frying pan and sauté the onion and garlic for 2 minutes.*
- *Stir in the Madeira and stock, and simmer gently for 2–3 minutes.*
- *Add the drained lentils and chickpeas to a small*

     *saucepan and heat through.*
- *Transfer the mixture to a blender, add the basil leaves, and purée.*

- *Place the sliced duck breast on pre-warmed plates, pour over the sauce and serve with the lentil purée.*
- *Season to taste and garnish with chopped chives.*

*Carbohydrate content per serving: **20** grams*

## Fresh trout with mustard and chive mayonnaise

For 2    2 large fresh trout fillets
25 grams butter, cubed
1 tbsp freshly squeezed orange juice
2 tbsp Mustard and chive mayonnaise (page 223)
Freshly ground black pepper
1 tbsp freshly chopped chives, to garnish

- *Place the trout fillets in an oven-safe dish, dot with butter, cover with pierced aluminium foil and cook in the centre of a preheated oven at 180°C (gas mark 4) for 18–20 minutes.*
- *Lay the trout fillets in the centre of the plates and drizzle over the orange juice.*
- *Spoon the Mustard and chive mayonnaise next to the trout, season to taste and garnish with freshly chopped chives.*
- *Serve immediately.*

*Carbohydrate content per serving: **2** grams*

**Barbary duck with teriyaki sauce**

The ingredients in this recipe may seem a little exotic, but actually all are available in most supermarkets – although a much wider variety is available in specialist delicatessens.

For 2
2 tbsp extra-virgin olive oil
2 medium Barbary duck breasts
25 grams butter, cubed
100 grams wild rocket leaves
Freshly ground black pepper

Teriyaki sauce
2 tbsp shohu (Japanese soy sauce)
2 tbsp sake
2 tbsp mirin (sweet Japanese wine)
1 tsp runny honey
2 slices root ginger, peeled and finely chopped
1 tbsp freshly squeezed lemon juice
1 tbsp chopped fresh coriander leaves

- *Heat the extra-virgin olive oil in a medium frying pan and sear the duck breasts for 4 minutes, turning once.*
- *Transfer the duck breast to an oven-safe dish, dot with cubed butter, cover with pierced aluminium foil and bake in the centre of a preheated oven at 180°C (gas mark 4) for 30 minutes, then set aside to cool for 10 minutes.*

*5 minutes before the duck breasts are ready*
- *Prepare the sauce. Heat the shohu, sake, mirin, honey, ginger, lemon juice and coriander in a medium saucepan for 2–3 minutes.*

- *Slice the duck breast and serve on a bed of rocket.*
- *Drizzle over the teriyaki sauce, season to taste with freshly ground black pepper and serve immediately.*

*Carbohydrate content per serving: **7** grams*

**Balti chicken with tzatziki**

For 2    2 tbsp extra-virgin olive oil
             2 medium chicken breasts, skin removed and sliced
             2 tbsp Balti spices, bought ready-made
             100 grams wild rocket
             150 ml Tzatziki (page 171)

- *Heat the extra-virgin olive oil in a wok and stir-fry the chicken for 3–4 minutes.*
- *Coat the chicken with the Balti spices and stir-fry for a further 2 minutes.*
- *Serve the Balti chicken on a bed of wild rocket and top with Tzatziki.*

*Carbohydrate content per serving: **16** grams*

**Sliced turkey with orange and basil**

For 2    2 tbsp extra-virgin olive oil

4 slices turkey breast, approximately 75 grams each

2 shallots, peeled and finely chopped

1 garlic clove, peeled and finely chopped

5 tbsp chicken stock

3 tbsp fresh orange juice

1 tsp fresh orange zest

1 tbsp chopped fresh basil

Freshly ground black pepper

2 pak choy, halved lengthways

- *Heat the extra-virgin olive oil in a medium frying pan and cook the turkey breast for 6–7 minutes, turning once.*
- *Remove the turkey from the pan with a slotted spoon and set aside.*
- *Add the shallots and garlic to the pan and sauté for 2–3 minutes.*
- *Return the turkey to the pan.*
- *Stir in the chicken stock, orange juice, orange zest and basil, and season to taste.*

*At the same time*
- *Lightly steam the pak choy for 4–5 minutes (or microwave on 'high' for 2–3 minutes).*

- *Serve the turkey with the pak choy and drizzle over the pan juices.*

*Carbohydrate content per serving: **7** grams*

**Chow mein**

This recipe includes prawns, but they can be substituted with 150 grams cooked chicken breast (finely sliced) or the shellfish can be omitted for a vegetarian version of the recipe.

For 2       60 grams Chinese egg noodles
150 grams peeled, cooked prawns
2 tbsp groundnut oil
100 grams bamboo shoots
75 grams mangetout (or Chinese cabbage, shredded)
2 slices of fresh ginger root, peeled and finely chopped
75 grams beansprouts
Few drops of sesame oil
Freshly ground black pepper
1 spring onion, finely chopped

Marinade

2 tbsp light soy sauce
1 tbsp rice wine or dry sherry
½ tsp cornflour
½ tsp caster sugar
1 tsp grated fresh ginger root

- *Add the Chinese egg noodles to 1½ litres of water in a large saucepan, stir in a teaspoon of rock salt and bring to the boil.*
- *Cook for 3–4 minutes then drain.*

*At the same time*
- *Mix together the marinade ingredients and marinate the prawns for 30–60 minutes.*

- *Heat the groundnut oil in a wok and stir-fry the*

bamboo shoots, mangetout and ginger for 1–2
minutes.
- Stir in the marinated prawns, beansprouts and
  sesame oil, then stir-fry for another 2 minutes.
- Stir in the noodles, heat through for a further minute,
  then season to taste and serve immediately,
  garnished with finely chopped spring onion.

*Carbohydrate content per serving: **30** grams*

**Scallops with lemon chilli**

For 2   6 fresh scallops
Juice of a fresh lemon
1 green chilli, finely chopped
1 tbsp chopped fresh mint leaves
Freshly ground black pepper
2 tbsp extra-virgin olive oil

- *Separate the orange corals from the scallops and slice the scallops into rounds horizontally.*
- *Mix together the scallops (and corals) with the lemon juice, chilli, mint and pepper, and marinate in the fridge for 1–2 hours.*
- *Heat the extra-virgin olive oil in a medium frying pan and sauté the scallops (and marinade) for 3–4 minutes, turning once.*
- *Serve immediately.*

*Carbohydrate content per serving: **2** grams*

**Warm spinach curry**

For 2    2 tbsp extra-virgin olive oil
1 large red onion, peeled and finely diced
1 medium garlic clove, peeled and finely chopped
½ tsp garam masala
½ tsp ground turmeric
¼ tsp ground fenugreek
1 tbsp chopped fresh coriander leaves
250 grams fresh spinach leaves

- *Heat the extra-virgin olive oil in a medium frying pan and sauté the onion and garlic for 2–3 minutes.*
- *Remove from the heat and stir in the garam masala, turmeric and fenugreek.*
- *Return to the heat and stir in the coriander and spinach.*
- *Stir-fry over a low heat until the spinach begins to wilt, and serve immediately.*

*Carbohydrate content per serving: **8** grams*

## Mussels with ginger and herbs

For 2    500 grams fresh mussels, debearded and scrubbed
1 tbsp groundnut oil
2 shallots, peeled and diced
1 large garlic clove, peeled and sliced
3 slices fresh ginger root, peeled and sliced into
   matchsticks
150 ml dry white wine
1 tbsp chopped flat-leaf parsley
1 tbsp ground almonds

- *Wash and scrub the mussels, discarding any that are open.*
- *Heat the groundnut oil in a medium saucepan and sauté the shallots and garlic for 1–2 minutes.*
- *Stir in the ginger, wine, parsley and almonds, then add the mussels.*
- *Bring to the boil, then cover the pan and simmer for 5–6 minutes.*
- *Serve immediately, discarding any unopened mussels.*

*Carbohydrate content per serving: **5** grams*

**Smoked salmon with horseradish and crème fraîche dressing**

For 2    100 grams smoked salmon, finely sliced

4 tbsp Horseradish and crème fraîche dressing (page 224)

75 grams French beans, topped and tailed

75 grams baby spinach leaves

1 Lebanese cucumber, chopped into matchsticks

Balsamic vinaigrette (page 222)

Freshly ground black pepper

- *Mix together the smoked salmon and Horseradish dressing, and set aside to cool in the fridge.*
- *Lightly steam the French beans for 4–5 minutes (or microwave on 'high' for 2–3 minutes), and allow to cool.*
- *Mix together the baby spinach, cucumber and French beans in a medium bowl and drizzle over a few drops of Balsamic vinaigrette.*
- *Serve the smoked salmon with Horseradish and crème fraîche dressing with a green salad, and season to taste.*

*Carbohydrate content per serving: **6** grams*

**Hot fettuccine with basil and chicken**

For 2
2 medium chicken breasts (about 150 grams each)
25 grams butter cubes
60 grams fettuccine, dry or fresh
2 tbsp extra-virgin olive oil
1 medium brown onion, peeled and chopped
50 grams button mushrooms, wiped and sliced
2 tbsp sun-dried tomatoes in extra-virgin olive oil,
    drained and finely sliced
1 tbsp chopped fresh basil leaves
4 green olives, finely sliced
1 tbsp Parmesan cheese, freshly grated
Freshly ground black pepper

Sauce
15 grams unsalted butter
2 tsp plain wholemeal flour
75 ml full-cream milk

- *Place the chicken breasts in an oven-safe dish, dot with butter cubes, cover with pierced aluminium foil and cook in the centre of a pre-heated oven at 180°C (gas mark 4) for 35–40 minutes.*
- *Remove from the oven. Set aside to cool, then slice finely.*

*Just before the chicken has cooked*
- *Place the pasta into a large pan of boiling water and cook for about 8 minutes (or fresh pasta for 3–4 minutes).*
- *Heat the extra-virgin olive oil in a medium frying pan and sauté the onion and mushrooms for 3–4 minutes.*

*And*

- *Prepare the sauce. Melt the butter in a medium saucepan, remove from the heat and stir in the flour to form a smooth roux.*
- *Return to the heat and add the milk, stirring constantly.*
- *As the sauce thickens, remove from the heat.*

- *Mix the fettuccine with the chicken, onion, mushrooms, sun-dried tomatoes and basil in a large bowl, then gently stir in the sauce.*
- *Serve immediately, garnished with olives and Parmesan cheese.*
- *Season to taste.*

*Carbohydrate content per serving: **30** grams*

**Chicken chop suey**

For 2    3 tbsp groundnut oil

200 grams chicken breast, sliced into thin strips

1 garlic clove, peeled and finely chopped

3 slices fresh ginger root, peeled and finely chopped

2 spring onions, chopped into 3–4 cm lengths on the diagonal

75 grams beansprouts

75 grams bamboo shoots, sliced into thin strips

50 grams button mushrooms, wiped and finely sliced

Freshly ground black pepper

Sauce

3 tbsp light soy sauce

2 tbsp dry sherry

1 tsp cornflour

1 tsp granulated sugar

1 tbsp water

- *Heat 2 tbsp groundnut oil in the wok and stir-fry the chicken for 3–4 minutes.*
- *Remove from the wok and set aside.*
- *Heat the remaining tbsp groundnut oil in the wok and stir-fry the garlic, ginger, spring onions, beansprouts, bamboo shoots and mushrooms for 2–3 minutes.*
- *Mix together the sauce ingredients and stir into the vegetables.*
- *Return the chicken to the wok and stir-fry for a final 2 minutes.*
- *Season to taste and serve immediately.*

*Carbohydrate content per serving: **12** grams*

**Fresh rainbow trout with caper butter**

For 2     2 medium trout fillets, approximately 150 grams each
50 grams unsalted butter
1 tbsp capers, drained and rinsed
75 grams fresh watercress
Freshly ground black pepper
Fresh coriander leaves, to garnish

- *Microwave the trout fillets on 'high' for 2–3 minutes (depending on the oven), or place in an oven-safe dish, dot with a little butter, cover with pierced aluminium foil and cook in the centre of a preheated oven at 180°C (gas mark 4) for 15 minutes.*

*At the same time*

- *Melt the butter in a small saucepan, stir in the capers and heat gently for 1–2 minutes.*

- *Serve the trout fillets on a bed of watercress, drizzle over the caper butter, season to taste and garnish with fresh coriander.*

*Carbohydrate content per serving: **3** grams*

**Milanese risotto**

For 2
2 tbsp extra-virgin olive oil
1 small red onion, peeled and finely chopped
1 medium garlic clove, peeled and finely chopped
1 medium red pepper, deseeded and chopped
1 medium yellow pepper, deseeded and chopped
2 slices fresh ginger root, peeled and finely chopped
60 grams Arborio rice
3 tbsp dry white wine
200 ml chicken (or vegetable) stock
½ tsp saffron powder
1 tbsp freshly grated Parmesan cheese
1 tbsp fresh chopped parsley
Freshly ground black pepper

- *Heat the extra-virgin olive oil in a medium frying pan and sauté the onion, garlic and peppers for 1–2 minutes.*
- *Stir in the ginger and rice and cook for 1 minute.*
- *Add the wine and simmer gently for 1 minute.*
- *Stir in the stock and saffron powder and simmer gently until the rice is cooked and most of the liquid is absorbed.*
- *Add the Parmesan cheese and cook for a further minute, then remove from the heat, season to taste with freshly ground black pepper and serve immediately, topped with fresh parsley.*

*Carbohydrate content per serving: **30** grams*

**Char-grilled swordfish with mustard dressing**

For 2
2 medium swordfish steaks, approximately 150 grams each
2 tbsp extra-virgin olive oil
1 pak choy, halved lengthways
Mustard vinaigrette (page 222)
Freshly ground black pepper

* *Brush the swordfish steaks with extra-virgin olive oil and grill under a hot grill (no closer than 8–10 cm from the grill) for 6–8 minutes, turning once.*

*At the same time*

* *Lightly steam the pak choy for 5–6 minutes (or microwave, in a microwave-safe container, for 2–3 minutes).*

* *Serve the swordfish steaks with the pak choy, drizzle over the Mustard vinaigrette and season to taste.*

*Carbohydrate content per serving: **3** grams*

**Cajun-style cod with fennel and herb salad**

For 2    2 tbsp extra-virgin olive oil
2 cod steaks, approximately 150 grams each
2 tsp Cajun seasoning, bought ready-made
Fennel and herb salad (page 193)
Freshly ground black pepper

- *Heat the extra-virgin olive oil in a medium saucepan.*
- *Coat one side of each cod steak with approximately ½ tsp Cajun seasoning, then fry, seasoned-side down, for about 2 minutes.*
- *Coat the upper surface of the steaks with another ½ tsp Cajun seasoning, then turn over and cook for a further 2–3 minutes.*
- *Season to taste and serve immediately with Fennel and herb salad.*

*Carbohydrate content per serving: **9** grams*

**Crunchy tiger prawn 'pie'**

For 2    6 large raw tiger prawns
2 tbsp wholegrain mustard
150 grams ground almonds
1 tbsp finely chopped fresh coriander
Large handful (approximately 50 grams) fresh baby
spinach leaves

- *Wash the tiger prawns, then pat dry.*
- *Coat the prawns with the wholegrain mustard.*
- *Mix the ground almonds with the coriander and roll the prawns in the mixture to coat thoroughly.*
- *Place on a baking tray in a single layer then cook in the centre of a preheated oven at 180°C (gas mark 4) for 7–8 minutes.*
- *Serve immediately on a bed of fresh baby spinach leaves.*

*Carbohydrate content per serving: 7 grams*

# Pasta

Contrary to popular belief (and misconceptions), pasta *can* be included in a healthy low-carb diet. However, it must be weighed carefully as it consists of approximately 70 per cent carbohydrate.

And the *shape* of the pasta is irrelevant; almost all shapes of pasta are made from the same recipe so they all contain approximately 70 per cent carbohydrate, whether it be spaghetti, fusilli, tagliatelli, macaroni, lasagne, linguine, penne, vermicelli, Hokkien noodles . . . or any of the other multiple variation of shapes and configurations of pasta and noodles. However, some types of egg noodles can be as low as 20 per cent carbohydrate – so remember to read the nutritional label!

The only form of pasta which has real nutritional benefits is wholemeal pasta; other varieties have had most (if not all) of the nutrition removed during the refining process. All of the following recipes incorporate wholemeal pasta for this reason, although obviously alternative pastas (with lesser nutritional benefit) can be used if you don't like the wholemeal variety.

The other important point to remember is that pasta increases to approximately two and a half times its dry weight when cooked, so 40 grams of *dried* pasta increases to about 100 grams of *cooked* pasta – more than sufficient for two people.

Many pasta dishes consist essentially of a pasta base with a relatively small amount of sauce stirred through the pasta. A more nutritious – and tasty – alternative is to reduce the volume of pasta, replacing the pasta with more nutritious ingredients.

## Easy pasta

For 2    1½ litres water
          Pinch of sea salt
          ½ tbsp extra-virgin olive oil
          40 grams dry wholemeal pasta

- *Boil the water in a large saucepan, then reduce the heat to a gentle simmer.*
- *Stir in the extra-virgin olive oil and salt, then add the pasta.*
- *Boil for 5 minutes, then remove from the heat and allow to stand for about 3 minutes.*
- *Drain the pasta and serve immediately.*

*Carbohydrate content per serving: **14** grams*

**Tagliatelli Carbonara**

For 2    40 grams dry wholemeal tagliatelli
1 fresh salmon steak (approximately 125–150 grams)
A little extra-virgin olive oil
100 ml double cream
40 grams freshly grated Parmesan
Freshly ground black pepper
1 tbsp freshly chopped flat-leaf parsley

- *Brush the salmon steak with extra-virgin olive oil.*
- *Grill the salmon for 6 minutes under a medium grill (no closer than 10 cm from the grill), turning once.*
- *Allow to cool for a few minutes, then flake the salmon steak, removing all bones and skin.*

*At the same time*
- *Cook the tagliatelli (page 126).*

*And*
- *Whisk the cream to slightly thicken.*

- *When the tagliatelli is cooked, transfer to a large, warm bowl and stir in the flaked salmon, cream and grated Parmesan.*
- *Season to taste then serve immediately, garnished with fresh parsley.*

*Carbohydrate content per serving: **16** grams*

### Wholemeal spaghetti Napolitana

For 2    2 tbsp extra-virgin olive oil
4 shallots, peeled and finely chopped
1 medium garlic clove, peeled and finely chopped
50 grams button mushrooms, wiped and sliced
   lengthways
440 grams tinned plum tomatoes
75 ml passata
1 tsp dried oregano
1 tsp dried basil
Pinch of salt
Freshly ground black pepper
40 grams wholemeal spaghetti

- *Heat the extra-virgin olive oil in a large frying pan and sauté the shallots and garlic for 2–3 minutes.*
- *Stir in the mushrooms and sauté for a further minute.*
- *Stir in the tomatoes, passata, oregano and basil, season to taste and simmer gently for 5–7 minutes.*

*At the same time*
- *Cook the spaghetti (page 126).*

- *When the spaghetti is cooked, stir in the Napolitana sauce and serve immediately.*

*Carbohydrate content per serving:* **26** *grams*

**Lasagne**

This meal has been prepared for four rather than two persons simply because we are constrained by the predetermined shape of the commercial sheets of lasagne. Of course, home-made lasagne can be easily made in smaller sizes and shapes.

For 4    Bolognese sauce (see page 131, but make enough for 4 servings)
30 grams unsalted butter
30 grams plain flour
150 ml milk
4 sheets of dried lasagne (60 grams carbohydrate)
1 tbsp freshly grated Parmesan cheese
100 grams fresh watercress
Balsamic vinegar
Freshly ground black pepper

- *Melt the butter in a medium saucepan, then remove from the heat and stir in the flour until the mixture is smooth.*
- *Return the pan to a gentle heat and gradually add the milk, stirring constantly, until the sauce just begins to thicken.*
- *Remove from the heat, continuing to stir.*
- *Using a roasting tin of approximately the same dimensions as the sheets of lasagne, spread about a quarter of the Bolognese sauce over the base of the tin, top with about a fifth of the white sauce, then cover with a sheet of lasagne.*
- *Repeat this three times, then cover the final sheet of lasagne with the remaining white sauce, sprinkle over the grated Parmesan cheese and cook in the centre of a preheated oven at 180°C (gas mark 4) for 30 minutes.*

- *Divide the lasagne into four equal portions and serve immediately with fresh watercress.*
- *Drizzle a little balsamic vinegar over the watercress and season to taste.*

*Carbohydrate content per serving: **20** grams*

**Spaghetti Bolognese**
Red meat is not essential for this most Italian of classical
dishes. Turkey mince is very nutritious and low in saturated fats
– or vegetarian mince can be substituted for the turkey mince,
and vegetable stock for the chicken stock for vegetarians.

For 2    Bolognese sauce
            3 tbsp extra-virgin olive oil
            1 medium red onion, peeled and chopped
            2 garlic cloves, peeled and finely chopped
            200 grams turkey mince (or vegetarian substitute)
            1 tbsp tomato purée
            150 ml chicken stock
            1 tbsp chopped fresh basil leaves (or 1 tsp dried basil)
            Freshly ground black pepper

            40 grams wholemeal spaghetti

- *Heat the extra-virgin olive oil in a medium frying pan.*
- *Sauté the onion and garlic for 2–3 minutes.*
- *Add the turkey mince and stir regularly until browned.*
- *Stir in the tomato purée, stock and basil, season to
  taste and simmer gently for 5–7 minutes.*

*At the same time*
- *Cook the spaghetti.*

- *When cooked, put the spaghetti in serving dishes
  and pour the sauce on top.*

*Carbohydrate content per serving: **20** grams*

### Penne with char-grilled vegetables

For 2    1 medium red onion, peeled and quartered
2 courgettes, chopped on the diagonal into 2–3 cm chunks
1 medium green pepper, deseeded and quartered
1 medium red pepper, deseeded and quartered
3 cherry tomatoes, halved
2 medium garlic cloves, peeled and finely chopped
2 tbsp extra-virgin olive oil
60 grams penne pasta
2 tbsp freshly grated Parmesan cheese
1 tbsp chopped fresh basil leaves
Freshly ground black pepper
Passata vinaigrette

- *Place the vegetables on a grill-safe, buttered baking tray, skin uppermost, sprinkling the chopped garlic over the vegetables.*
- *Drizzle with the extra-virgin olive oil and grill under a medium grill (no closer than 8–10 cm from the grill) for 5–7 minutes, turning twice.*
- *Remove from the heat and allow to cool for 1–2 minutes, then peel the skin from the peppers and tomatoes. Slice the peppers thinly.*

*At the same time*
- *Cook the penne pasta al dente.*

- *Stir the vegetables, Parmesan cheese and chopped basil into the pasta, season to taste with freshly ground black pepper, drizzle over a little Passata vinaigrette and serve immediately.*

*Carbohydrate content per serving: **29** grams*

**Fettuccine with spinach and sage**

For 2     60 grams fettuccine
2 tbsp extra-virgin olive oil
3 shallots, peeled and diced
2 medium garlic cloves, peeled and finely chopped
1 tbsp unsalted butter
100 grams chopped fresh spinach leaves
1 tbsp chopped fresh sage (or basil)
1 tbsp freshly grated Pecorino cheese
Freshly ground black pepper

- *Heat the extra-virgin olive oil in a small frying pan and sauté the shallots and garlic for 1–2 minutes.*
- *Melt the butter in a medium saucepan and cook the spinach and sage (or basil) for 30–60 seconds until it just begins to soften, then remove from the heat immediately.*

*At the same time*
- *Cook the fettuccine al dente.*

- *Stir the shallots, garlic, spinach, sage and Pecorino cheese into the fettuccine, season with freshly ground black pepper and serve immediately.*

*Carbohydrate content per serving: **25** grams*

**Angel hair pasta with capers and chilli**

For 2    2 tbsp groundnut oil
1 medium red onion, peeled and finely chopped
1 medium garlic clove, peeled and finely chopped
1 small green chilli, finely chopped (optional)
2 slices fresh ginger root, peeled and finely chopped
200 grams tinned peeled plum tomatoes
1 tbsp capers, drained and rinsed
1 tsp dried oregano
60 grams angel hair pasta
2 tbsp freshly grated Parmesan cheese
Freshly ground black pepper
1 tbsp freshly chopped chives (optional)

- *Heat the groundnut oil in a medium frying pan and sauté the onion and garlic for 1–2 minutes.*
- *Stir in the chilli, ginger, tomatoes, capers and oregano, and simmer gently for 8–10 minutes.*

*At the same time*
- *Cook the angel hair pasta for 3–4 minutes al dente.*

- *Stir the chilli mixture and the Parmesan cheese into the angel hair pasta, season to taste with freshly ground black pepper, garnish with freshly chopped chives and serve immediately.*

*Carbohydrate content per serving: **29** grams*

**Pappardelle with two-cheese sauce**

For 2    50 grams sun-dried tomatoes
50 grams freshly grated Parmesan cheese
1 tbsp ricotta cheese
1 tbsp fresh chopped coriander leaves
1 tbsp fresh chopped basil leaves
2 tbsp extra-virgin olive oil
60 grams pappardelle
Freshly ground black pepper

- *Blend together the tomatoes, Parmesan and ricotta cheese, coriander, basil and extra-virgin olive oil.*
- *Cook the pappardelle until al dente.*
- *Drain the pappardelle, stir through the sauce and heat gently for 1–2 minutes, then season to taste and serve immediately.*

*Carbohydrate content per serving: **25** grams*

**Tagliatelli with prawn and herb sauce**
Vegetarians can simply omit the prawns to enjoy a similarly
delicious meal.

For 2    25 grams unsalted butter
         25 grams plain flour
         150 ml milk
         100 grams cooked prawns, rinsed
         1 tbsp chopped fresh basil
         1 tbsp chopped fresh parsley
         50 grams tagliatelli
         Freshly ground black pepper
         1 spring onion, finely chopped

- *Melt the butter in a medium saucepan.*
- *Remove from the heat and stir in the flour.*
- *Return to a gentle heat and gradually add the milk, stirring constantly.*
- *When the mixture just begins to thicken, remove from the heat and stir in the prawns, basil and parsley.*

*At the same time*
- *Cook the tagliatelle al dente.*

- *Stir the sauce into the tagliatelle, season to taste with freshly ground black pepper and serve immediately, garnished with finely chopped spring onion.*

*Carbohydrate content per serving: **29 grams***

## Oven-baked mackerel with herb butter

For 2    50 grams unsalted butter
1 tbsp chopped fresh basil
1 tbsp chopped fresh coriander
1 tbsp freshly squeezed lemon juice
2 large fresh mackerel, gutted and cleaned
Freshly ground black pepper
Cucumber and radish salad

- *Heat the butter in a small saucepan until just melted, then stir in the basil, coriander and lemon juice.*
- *Score the mackerel several times on one surface, then pour the herb butter mixture into the cavity and scores along the fish.*
- *Season to taste with freshly ground black pepper.*
- *Wrap loosely in aluminium foil and cook in the centre of a preheated oven at 180°C (gas mark 4) for 25–30 minutes.*
- *Serve immediately with a cucumber and radish salad.*

*Carbohydrate content per serving: **20** grams*

**Wasabi tofu**

For 2    150 grams tofu, cubed
         2 tbsp extra-virgin olive oil
         50 grams mangetout
         50 grams sugar-snap peas
         Freshly ground black pepper

**Marinade**

         2 tsp wasabi paste (Japanese horseradish – very
            strong)
         2 tbsp shoyu (Japanese soy sauce)
         2 tbsp sake
         2 tbsp mirin
         2 slices root ginger, peeled and finely chopped
         Pinch of caster sugar
         1 tsp freshly ground black pepper

- *Mix together the wasabi paste, shoyu, sake, mirin,
  ginger, sugar and pepper in a medium mixing bowl
  and marinate the tofu for 3–4 hours.*
- *Heat the extra-virgin olive oil in a wok and stir-fry the
  tofu for 3–4 minutes.*

*At the same time*

- *Lightly steam the mangetout and sugar-snap peas for
  4–5 minutes, or microwave on high for 2–3 minutes.*

- *Serve the tofu on a bed of mangetout and sugar-snap
  peas and season to taste with freshly ground black
  pepper.*

*Carbohydrate content per serving: **8** grams*

**Fresh skate fillets with pepper sauce**

For 2    2 skate wings
50 grams unsalted butter, cubed
1 small yellow pepper, deseeded and finely sliced
1 small red pepper, deseeded and finely sliced
½ tbsp green peppercorns
100 ml single cream
1 tbsp freshly squeezed lemon juice
Fresh flat-leaf parsley, to garnish

- *Place the skate fillets in an oven-safe dish, dot with 25 grams of the butter (cubed), cover with pierced aluminium foil and bake in the centre of a preheated oven at 180°C (gas mark 4) for 15–20 minutes.*

*Just before the skate is cooked*
- *Melt the remaining butter in a medium frying pan and sauté the peppers and peppercorns for 2–3 minutes.*
- *Stir in the cream and lemon juice, lay the skate fillets in the pan and simmer very gently for 1 minute. Do not allow the cream to boil.*

- *Serve immediately, garnished with fresh flat-leaf parsley.*

*Carbohydrate content per serving: **7** grams*

## Button mushroom and basil risotto

For 2    2 tbsp groundnut oil
1 small brown onion, peeled and finely chopped
1 medium garlic clove, peeled and finely chopped
100 grams button mushrooms, wiped and halved
    vertically
60 grams Arborio rice
200 ml chicken (or vegetable) stock
1 tbsp fresh chopped basil leaves
1 tbsp fresh chopped mint leaves
Freshly ground black pepper

- *Heat the groundnut oil in a medium frying pan then sauté the onion and garlic for 1–2 minutes.*
- *Add the mushrooms and stir-fry for 3–4 minutes.*
- *Stir in the rice and add the stock.*
- *Simmer over a gentle heat for 8–10 minutes, stirring frequently, then stir in the basil and mint leaves.*
- *Simmer gently for a further 6–8 minutes until the rice is cooked, then season to taste with freshly ground black pepper and serve immediately.*

*Carbohydrate content per serving: **26** grams*

**Fillets of Dover sole with creamy mushroom sauce**

For 2    2 Dover sole fillets, approximately 150 grams each
100 ml dry white wine
20 grams unsalted butter
100 ml single cream
1 tsp cornflour
75 grams chestnut mushrooms, wiped and finely sliced
Freshly ground black pepper
Crispy green salad

- *Place the sole in an oven-safe dish, pour over the wine, cover with pierced aluminium foil and cook in the centre of a preheated oven at 180°C (gas mark 4) for 20 minutes.*

*At the same time*

- *Mix together the butter, cream and cornflour in a small bowl.*

- *When the sole has cooked, drain the liquid into a medium saucepan.*
- *Stir in the cornflour mixture and bring to the boil gently, stirring constantly.*
- *Add the mushrooms and cook for 1–2 minutes.*
- *Place the fish in the centre of the plates, pour over the mushroom sauce and season to taste.*
- *Serve with a crispy green salad.*

*Carbohydrate content per serving: **12** grams*

## Spicy crab with mango

For 2
150 grams fresh white crab meat
1 small red chilli, deseeded and finely chopped
½ small mango, chopped into 2 cm cubes
1 tbsp fresh chopped coriander leaves
50 grams unsalted butter
100 grams fresh spinach leaves
Freshly ground black pepper
Coriander leaves, to garnish

- *Mix together the crab meat, chilli, mango and chopped coriander leaves in a medium bowl.*
- *Melt the butter in a medium saucepan and cook the spinach leaves for 1 minute, or until just beginning to soften, stirring constantly.*
- *Serve the crab mixture on a bed of wilted spinach, season to taste and garnish with fresh coriander leaves.*

*Carbohydrate content per serving: **12** grams*

**Mussels with fontina and olive salad**

For 2   500 grams fresh mussels, debearded and scrubbed
Fontina and olive salad (page 195)
Lemon vinaigrette (page 221)
Freshly ground black pepper

- *Wash and scrub the mussels several times, discarding any that are open.*
- *Place the mussels in a large saucepan, add 4 tbsp water and bring to the boil.*
- *Simmer the mussels for 5–7 minutes until they open, discarding any that remain closed.*
- *Serve the mussels with Fontina and olive salad, drizzle over the Lemon vinaigrette and season to taste.*

*Carbohydrate content per serving: **6** grams*

**Ginger mushrooms and tofu with herb butter**

For 2    2 tbsp extra-virgin olive oil

2 shallots, peeled and diced

1 garlic clove, peeled and finely chopped

100 grams mixed mushrooms (chestnut, brown, button), wiped

100 grams tofu, cubed

2 slices of fresh ginger root, peeled and finely chopped

75 grams unsalted butter

1 tbsp chopped fresh basil

1 tbsp chopped fresh coriander

Freshly ground black pepper

- *Heat the extra-virgin olive oil in a medium frying pan and sauté the shallots and garlic for 2–3 minutes.*
- *Stir in the mushrooms, tofu and ginger, and stir-fry for 3–4 minutes.*

*At the same time*

- *Melt the butter in a medium saucepan and stir in the basil and coriander. Do not overheat!*

- *Serve the herb butter over the mushrooms and tofu, and season to taste.*

*Carbohydrate content per serving: **4** grams*

## Smoked haddock kedgeree

For 2    2 medium smoked haddock fillets (approximately
         150 grams each)
         25 grams unsalted butter, cubed
         50 grams wholegrain rice
         2 tbsp extra-virgin olive oil
         1 medium red onion, peeled and chopped
         ½ tsp medium curry powder
         1 large free-range hard-boiled egg, peeled and chopped
         1 tbsp chopped fresh basil
         1 tbsp chopped fresh parsley
         Freshly ground black pepper

- *Place the haddock fillets in a medium, oven-safe baking dish, dot with butter and cover with pierced aluminium foil.*
- *Cook in the centre of a preheated oven at 180°C (gas mark 4) for 20 minutes, then remove from the heat and flake the haddock.*

*At the same time*
- *Cook the rice.*

- *Heat the extra-virgin olive oil in a medium frying pan and sauté the onion for 1–2 minutes.*
- *Stir in the curry powder and cook for a few seconds, then stir in the cooked rice, egg, flaked haddock, basil and parsley.*
- *Cook over a gentle heat for 2–3 minutes, then season to taste and serve immediately.*

*Carbohydrate content per serving: **20** grams*

**Chilli con carne**

This recipe is equally suitable for vegetarians by substituting
turkey mince with vegetarian mince, and chicken stock with
vegetable stock. It is just as delicious without the chilli for those
averse to hot dishes.

For 2    30 grams dried red kidney beans (or 50 grams tinned
              red kidney beans)
         2 tbsp extra-virgin olive oil
         1 medium red onion, peeled and chopped
         200 grams turkey mince
         1 level tbsp wholemeal flour
         ½ tsp chilli powder (optional)
         1 tbsp tomato purée
         200 ml chicken stock
         50 grams wholegrain rice

- *Place the dried kidney beans in a medium saucepan,
  cover with cold water and bring to the boil for 15
  minutes, then remove from the heat and allow to cool
  for at least 1 hour.*
- *Drain the cooked (or tinned) beans.*
- *Heat the extra-virgin olive oil in a medium frying pan
  and sauté the onion and garlic for 1–2 minutes.*
- *Add the mince and cook until brown.*
- *Stir in the flour, chilli powder and tomato purée, then
  gradually add the stock.*
- *Simmer gently for 10 minutes.*

*At the same time*
- *Cook the rice.*

- *When cooked, serve the chilli with the rice.*

*Carbohydrate content per serving: **31** grams*

As mentioned at the beginning of the chapter, there are many other delicious red meat-free recipes described in the other books in this series. Of course, this list only includes recipes incorporating either seafood or poultry; the pure vegetarian recipes in previous books are listed in Chapter 11.

## The New High Protein Diet Cookbook

- Chicken Marsala
- Chilli tiger prawns
- Tarragon chicken
- Trout with watercress and mint sauce
- Chicken with creamy curry mayonnaise
- Calamari and ginger
- Roast chicken with broccoli
- Spiced turkey kebabs
- Trout with mustard cream sauce
- Lobster with basil and chive sauce
- Turkey with rosemary and thyme
- Smoked trout pâté
- Cod kebabs with baby squash
- Chicken cacciatore
- Citrus cod and rocket
- Spicy Thai swordfish
- Cod with chive and parsley butter sauce
- Turkey curry with almonds
- Spicy haddock with stir-fried vegetables
- Chilli prawn soufflé
- Chicken paprika
- Salmon steaks with herbs
- Honey and ginger chicken
- Salmon and basil pâté
- Spicy tiger prawns with coconut
- Chicken with macadamia nuts

- Chilli prawns with coriander
- Teriyaki salmon
- Chicken with mushroom casserole
- Crab with herbs
- Whiting with spicy batter
- Creamy smoked haddock pâté
- Tuna and oregano casserole
- Cheese and chives soufflé
- Swordfish steaks with asparagus
- Smoked mackerel pâté
- Taramasalata
- Swordfish with mustard and honey
- Salmon with herbs
- Tuna and salmon sashimi
- Smoked haddock with prawns
- Cod and basil casserole
- Cod with coriander
- Chilli scallops
- Cod with olive and caper sauce
- Prawn fu-yung
- Coconut chicken with pine nuts
- Crab with crème fraîche
- Chicken chop suey
- Pepper haddock with mustard sauce
- Scallops with honey and orange vinaigrette
- Herb chicken burgers
- Tiger prawns with ginger and garlic
- Peppered salmon steaks with lime
- Chicken and ginger
- Calamari with basil and coriander
- Piperade
- Salmon with bok choy
- Crab with spicy mayonnaise

- Poached whiting with ginger
- Chilli turkey
- Oysters au natural
- Tuna with bok choy
- Soufflé omelette
- Char-grilled tuna steaks
- Shellfish omelette

## The New High Protein Healthy Fast Food Diet

- Salmon with lime butter sauce and watercress
- Spicy chicken drumsticks
- Duck with plum sauce
- Mint cod with rocket and spinach
- Chicken satay with lime
- Thai chicken with lemongrass and ginger
- Chicken korma with mangetout and broccoli
- Turkey teriyaki
- Prawn omelette
- Turkey in cherry tomato and chilli sauce
- Turkey bolognaise with peppers
- Spicy scrambled eggs
- Salmon with Bocconcini and basil
- Peking duck
- Plaice with olives
- Balti chicken
- Eggs Benedict
- Mozzarella and tomato omelette
- Salmon with wild rocket and mint sauce
- Peppered smoked mackerel with spinach in butter sauce
- Bombay turkey breast with watercress and rocket salad
- Chargrilled basil pesto salmon with asparagus

# Chapter 11 Vegetarian meals and salads

One of the commonest misconceptions regarding a healthy low-carb diet is that it cannot be followed by vegetarians. It is often misrepresented as a diet which is essentially based on meat. In some low-carb diets this is true – but it is certainly not an essential prerequisite of a healthy low-carb diet. As you can see from the previous chapters of this book, nothing could be further from the truth! There are no red meat products included in this diet. Even if one wished to exclude fish, shellfish, poultry and eggs, it is still possible to follow a healthy, low-GI/low-carb diet – although, as previously mentioned, if you exclude all animal-based products from your diet you must take regular vitamin $B^{12}$ supplements as this vitamin is not present in foods of exclusively plant origin.

This book contains 38 main meals suitable for vegetarians, 22 side dishes and 9 salads, with information on an additional 37 delicious salads described in previous books in the series. This is merely the tiniest fraction of vegetarian meals suitable for inclusion in a healthy low-GI/low-carb diet. In fact, it is intended to provide you with the principles of adapting this diet to the many different types of suitable vegetarian foods, because the inclusion of fresh vegetables in good quantities is absolutely essential for any healthy diet.

# Vegetarian main meals

Many of the recipes described in earlier chapters are equally suitable for vegetarians. These include:

Chestnut mushrooms with herb butter

Tomato and aubergine soup

Hearty pumpkin and tomato soup

Creamy mushroom soup

Spicy tomato and lentil soup

Hot and spicy tomato soup

Mascarpone and spinach soup

Mulligatawny soup

Chilled cucumber soup

Tofu and red pepper soup

Angel hair pasta with Italian sauce

Penne rigate with mixed veggies

Stir-fried tofu with mushrooms

Coconut okra curry

Chow mein

Warm spinach curry

Milanese risotto

Wholemeal spaghetti Napolitana

Lasagne

Penne with chargrilled vegetables

Fettuccine with spinach and sage

Angel hair pasta with capers and chilli

Wasabi tofu

Button mushroom and basil risotto

Ginger mushrooms and tofu with herb butter

Pappardelle with two-cheese sauce

Chilli con carne (vegetarian version)

**Mozzarella aubergine slices with pesto sauce**

For 2     1 large aubergine, washed and sliced finely lengthways
Sea salt
3 tbsp extra-virgin olive oil
1 medium garlic clove, peeled and finely chopped
2 tbsp coriander pesto sauce
75 grams mozzarella cheese, sliced very finely
Freshly ground black pepper
1 tbsp chopped fresh chives
Fresh coriander leaves, washed

- *Place the aubergine slices in a colander, sprinkle with salt and leave for 20–30 minutes. Rinse with cold water and pat dry.*
- *Heat the extra-virgin olive oil in a large, shallow frying pan, then lightly fry the aubergine slices and garlic for 2–3 minutes, turning once.*
- *Spoon the pesto sauce evenly on each of the aubergine slices, top with the finely sliced mozzarella and grill under a hot grill (no closer than 8–10 cm from the grill) for 3–4 minutes, or until the mozzarella just begins to 'bubble'.*
- *Serve the mozzarella aubergine slices on warmed plates, season to taste and garnish with chopped fresh chives and coriander leaves.*

*Carbohydrate content per serving: **6** grams*

### Spicy carrot and coriander patties

For 2
2 large carrots, peeled and grated
2 shallots, peeled and finely chopped
2 slices of fresh ginger root, peeled and grated
1 small garlic clove, peeled and grated
1 tbsp chopped fresh coriander leaves
1 tbsp freshly grated Parmesan cheese
1 tbsp Bombay crushed curry spices, bought ready-made
1 tbsp plain flour
1 medium organic free-range egg, beaten
2 tbsp extra-virgin olive oil
Pinch of rock salt
Freshly ground black pepper
100 grams wild rocket
Sprigs of fresh mint, to garnish

- *Mix together the carrots, shallots, ginger, garlic, coriander, Parmesan cheese, spices and flour in a large bowl.*
- *Stir in the beaten egg.*
- *Form the carrot mixture into small patties.*
- *Heat the extra-virgin olive oil in a large frying pan.*
- *Cook the patties for 3–4 minutes, turning once.*
- *Season to taste and serve immediately with wild rocket and sprigs of fresh mint.*

*Carbohydrate content per serving: **15** grams*

### Char-grilled tofu kebabs with satay sauce

For 2   75 grams tofu, chopped into 2 cm cubes
50 grams small button mushrooms, wiped
1 small green pepper, deseeded and chopped into
     2 cm cubes
1 small red pepper, deseeded and chopped into
     2 cm cubes
6 small yellow squash, halved lengthways
Freshly ground black pepper
1 tbsp chopped fresh basil leaves
Satay sauce (page 225)

### Marinade

2 tbsp soy sauce
2 tbsp dry sherry
2 slices of fresh root ginger, peeled and grated
1 small garlic clove, peeled and grated

- *Mix together the ingredients of the marinade and marinate the cubed tofu for 3–4 hours.*

### At the same time

- *Soak the satay sticks in cold water.*

- *Thread the tofu, mushrooms, peppers and squash alternately onto the satay sticks.*
- *Drizzle over the remaining marinade and cook under a hot grill (no closer than 8–10 cm from the grill) for 6–8 minutes, turning frequently.*
- *Season to taste, garnish with chopped fresh basil leaves and serve with Satay sauce.*

*Carbohydrate content per serving: **27** grams*

### Classic macaroni cheese

A classic recipe which can be incorporated into a nutritious, low-carb diet.

For 2    30 grams unsalted butter
30 grams wholemeal flour
½ tsp mustard powder
150 ml full-cream milk
40 grams Cheddar cheese, grated
1 tbsp chopped fresh basil leaves
1 tbsp chopped fresh flat-leaf parsley
Freshly ground black pepper
50 grams organic macaroni
100 grams fresh wild rocket leaves

- *Melt the butter in a medium saucepan and stir in the flour and mustard powder.*
- *Remove from the heat and gradually add the milk, stirring constantly.*
- *Return to a moderate heat, stirring constantly, until the mixture just begins to thicken.*
- *Stir in the cheese, basil leaves and flat-leaf parsley, and season to taste.*

*At the same time*
- *Cook the macaroni in a large saucepan of boiling water for 8–10 minutes, then drain.*

- *Stir the macaroni into the sauce and serve immediately with fresh wild rocket.*

*Carbohydrate content per serving: **34** grams*

**Baby spinach with sesame seeds**

For 2    40 grams unsalted butter
3 spring onions, chopped on the diagonal into
    2–3 cm lengths
1 medium garlic clove, peeled and finely chopped
50 grams chestnut mushrooms, wiped and sliced
75 grams baby spinach leaves, washed
6 cherry tomatoes on-the-vine, halved
2 slices of fresh ginger root, peeled and finely chopped
1 tsp freshly squeezed lemon juice
1 tsp soy sauce
1 tsp dry sherry
Freshly ground black pepper
2 tsp sesame seeds

- *Melt the butter in a medium frying pan and sauté the spring onions, garlic and mushrooms for 2–3 minutes, stirring constantly.*
- *Stir in the baby spinach leaves, cherry tomatoes, ginger, lemon juice, soy sauce and sherry, and season to taste.*
- *Dry stir-fry the sesame seeds for 1 minute.*
- *Serve the stir-fried spinach immediately, and sprinkle the toasted sesame seeds on top.*

*Carbohydrate content per serving: **9** grams*

## Ratatouille

There are many variations on this traditional French dish, one of which has appeared in a previous book! Here is a delicious variation, which is quick and nutritious.

For 2      1 medium ripe aubergine, chopped into 2–3 cm cubes
           Sea salt
           3 tbsp extra-virgin olive oil
           1 medium red onion, peeled and chopped
           1 medium garlic clove, peeled and chopped
           2 medium courgettes, sliced
           1 medium red pepper, deseeded and sliced
           1 medium yellow pepper, deseeded and sliced
           440 grams tinned plum tomatoes
           1 tsp dried oregano
           1 tsp dried basil
           Pinch of sea salt
           Freshly ground black pepper

- *Place the cubed aubergine in a colander, sprinkle with sea salt and allow to stand for 30 minutes. Rinse with cold water and pat dry.*
- *Heat the extra-virgin olive oil in a large frying pan and sauté the onion and garlic for 1–2 minutes.*
- *Add the aubergine, courgettes and peppers, and stir-fry for 4–5 minutes.*
- *Stir in the tomatoes and herbs, season to taste and gently simmer for 20–25 minutes.*

*Carbohydrate content per serving: **19** grams*

## Lentil dhal

For 2    200 grams brown lentils
2 tbsp extra-virgin olive oil
1 medium red onion, peeled and finely chopped
1 small garlic clove, peeled and crushed
1 large green chilli, deseeded and finely chopped
½ tsp ground coriander
½ tsp ground cumin
¼ tsp chilli powder
½ tsp garam masala
¼ tsp ground turmeric
600 ml organic vegetable stock

- *Place lentils in a medium bowl, cover with cold water and allow to stand for at least 8 hours, then drain before use.*
- *Heat the extra-virgin olive oil in a medium saucepan and sauté the onion and garlic for 1–2 minutes.*
- *Stir in the chilli, coriander, cumin, chilli powder, garam masala and turmeric, and stir-fry for a further 2 minutes.*
- *Stir in the vegetable stock and lentils, and simmer gently for about 1 hour.*
- *Serve immediately.*

*Carbohydrate content per serving: **24** grams*

### Ricotta soufflé

For 2   30 grams unsalted butter
1½ tbsp wholemeal flour
Pinch of dry mustard powder
150 ml full-cream milk
75 grams Ricotta cheese, crumbled
3 large organic free-range eggs, separated
2 tsp freshly grated Parmesan cheese
Freshly ground black pepper

- *Heat the butter in a medium saucepan and stir in the flour and mustard to form a roux.*
- *Remove from the heat and gradually add the milk, stirring frequently.*
- *Return to the heat, stirring constantly, until the mixture just begins to thicken.*
- *Remove from the heat and stir in the cheese and egg yolks.*
- *Beat the egg whites in a medium mixing bowl, then gradually fold the egg whites into the mixture.*
- *Pour the mixture into a soufflé dish and sprinkle over the Parmesan cheese.*
- *Cook in the centre of a preheated oven at 180°C (gas mark 4) for about 20–25 minutes, season to taste and serve immediately.*

*Carbohydrate content per serving: **15** grams*

**Garlic aubergine with tabbouleh**

For 2
1 medium aubergine, peeled and chopped
Sea salt
3 tbsp extra-virgin olive oil
1 small garlic clove, peeled and grated
Pinch of cayenne pepper
40 grams Tabbouleh (page 170)
Red lettuce salad

- *Place the cubed aubergine in a colander, sprinkle with sea salt and allow to stand for 30 minutes. Rinse with cold water and pat dry.*
- *Heat the extra-virgin olive oil in a large frying pan and stir-fry the aubergine, garlic and cayenne pepper for about 5 minutes.*
- *Transfer the aubergine cubes to warm plates.*
- *Serve immediately with Tabbouleh and a red lettuce salad.*

*Carbohydrate content per serving: **28** grams*

## Baked pepper frittata

Chillis are members of the capsicum (or 'pepper') family, so this is truly a 'pepper' frittata.

For 2

2 tbsp extra-virgin olive oil
1 small red onion, peeled and chopped
1 small garlic clove, peeled and finely chopped
½ small yellow pepper, deseeded and finely chopped
½ small red pepper, deseeded and finely chopped
1 small red chilli, deseeded and finely chopped
Freshly ground black pepper
1 tbsp chopped fresh basil leaves
3 large fresh organic free-range eggs, beaten
100 ml single cream
100 grams Red Leicester cheese, grated
1 tbsp freshly grated Parmesan cheese
Green salad with herbs

- *Heat the extra-virgin olive oil in a medium frying pan and sauté the onion and garlic for 2–3 minutes.*
- *Add the peppers and chilli, season to taste and stir-fry for 2–3 minutes.*
- *Mix together the basil leaves, eggs and cream.*
- *Grease a medium, deep baking dish, spoon a layer of pepper mixture in the base, top with a thin layer of egg mixture and sprinkle over some cheese.*
- *Alternate thin layers of pepper mixture, egg mixture and cheese.*
- *Top with a layer of freshly grated Parmesan cheese and bake in the centre of a preheated oven at 180°C (gas mark 4) for 20–25 minutes.*
- *Serve immediately with a green salad with herbs.*

*Carbohydrate content per serving: **8** grams*

**Nasi Goreng**

For 2    60 grams Arborio rice
25 grams unsalted butter
2 large free-range eggs, beaten
2 tbsp extra-virgin olive oil
2 shallots, peeled and chopped
1 garlic clove, peeled and chopped
1 slice of fresh ginger root, peeled and chopped
1 medium green chilli, peeled and finely chopped
1 medium red pepper, deseeded and finely sliced
1 medium orange pepper, deseeded and finely sliced
2 spring onions, chopped on the diagonal into
   2–3 cm lengths
1 tbsp chopped fresh coriander leaves
1 tbsp chopped fresh basil leaves
1 tbsp soy sauce
Freshly ground black pepper
100 grams fresh wild rocket

- *Cook the rice.*

*Just before the rice is cooked*
- *Heat the butter in a medium pan and scramble the eggs, stirring constantly, then set aside.*
- *Heat the extra-virgin olive oil in a wok and stir-fry the shallots, garlic, ginger, chilli, peppers, spring onions, coriander and basil for 2–3 minutes.*

- *Stir in the scrambled eggs, cooked rice and soy sauce and stir-fry for a further minute.*
- *Season to taste and serve immediately on a bed of wild rocket.*

*Carbohydrate content per serving: **30** grams*

# Vegetable side-dishes

**Courvoisier mushrooms with cream**

For 2
2 tbsp extra-virgin olive oil
3 shallots, peeled and chopped
1 garlic clove, peeled and chopped
150 grams chestnut mushrooms, wiped
1 tbsp Courvoisier brandy (optional)
40 ml single cream
1 tbsp chopped fresh basil leaves
Freshly ground black pepper

• *Heat the extra-virgin olive oil in a medium frying pan and gently sauté the shallots and garlic for 2–3 minutes.*
• *Add the mushrooms and stir-fry over a medium heat for 3–4 minutes.*
• *Stir in the brandy, cream and basil, and heat through gently for 1–2 minutes.*
• *Season to taste and serve immediately.*

*Carbohydrate content per serving: **6 grams***

**Harissa**

For 2
3 large garlic cloves, skin removed
2 medium red peppers, deseeded and finely sliced
3 medium red chillis, sliced
2 tbsp extra-virgin olive oil
1 tsp cumin seeds
1 tsp coriander seeds

- *Place the garlic cloves on a baking tray, then bake in the centre of a preheated oven at 180°C (gas mark 4) for 40–50 minutes.*
- *Open the garlic cloves and remove the soft garlic pulp for later use.*

*At the same time*
- *Sauté the peppers and chillis in 1 tbsp of the extra-virgin olive oil for about 8–10 minutes.*
- *Dry-roast the cumin and coriander seeds in a medium frying pan for 1 minutes.*

- *Place the garlic, peppers, chillis, cumin and coriander seeds in a blender, add the remaining 1 tbsp of olive oil and blend.*

*Carbohydrate content per serving: **7** grams*

**Oriental shredded chilli cabbage**

For 2  ½ medium red cabbage (approx 250 grams), finely
sliced
1 tsp sea salt
1 tbsp extra-virgin olive oil
2 tsp sesame oil
2 shallots, peeled and finely chopped
2 spring onions, sliced on the diagonal into 3–4 cm
lengths
1 small red chilli, finely chopped (optional)
2 slices of fresh ginger root, peeled and finely chopped
2 tsp granulated sugar
30 ml water
1 tbsp white wine vinegar
Freshly ground black pepper

- *Place the sliced cabbage in a colander and sprinkle
with salt. Allow to stand for 30–40 minutes, then
rinse with cold water and pat dry.*
- *Heat the extra-virgin olive oil and sesame oil in a wok
and stir-fry the shallots, spring onions, chilli and
ginger for 1–2 minutes.*
- *Stir in the sugar and water for about 30 seconds,
then add the white wine vinegar.*
- *Add the cabbage and stir-fry for 2–3 minutes, season
to taste and serve immediately.*

*Carbohydrate content per serving: **11** grams*

**Root vegetables with asparagus and chive sour cream**

For 2   ½ small swede, peeled and cubed
1 small carrot, peeled and chopped
Pinch of grated nutmeg
8 asparagus spears, washed
1 tbsp freshly chopped chives
100 ml soured cream
Freshly ground black pepper

- *Lightly steam the swede and carrot for 7–8 minutes, or microwave on high for 3–4 minutes.*
- *Mash together the swede and carrot, adding a pinch of nutmeg.*

*At the same time*
- *Lightly steam the asparagus for 4–5 minutes, or microwave on high for 3–4 minutes.*

*And*
- *Stir the chopped chives into the soured cream.*

- *Serve the asparagus on a bed of mashed swede and carrot.*
- *Top with chive soured cream.*
- *Season to taste with freshly ground black pepper and serve immediately.*

*Carbohydrate content per serving: **7 grams***

**Cheesy baked tomatoes with black olives**

For 2   2 large beefsteak tomatoes.
2 tbsp extra-virgin olive oil
2 shallots, peeled and finely chopped
1 medium garlic clove, peeled and finely chopped
6 black olives, pitted
25 grams button mushrooms, wiped and finely sliced
1 tbsp freshly grated Parmesan cheese
1 tbsp chopped fresh basil
Freshly ground black pepper

- *Cut the tops off the tomatoes and remove the seeds.*
- *Heat the extra-virgin olive oil in a medium saucepan and sauté the shallots, garlic, olives and mushrooms for 2 minutes.*
- *Stir in the Parmesan cheese and basil, and season to taste.*
- *Spoon the mixture into the tomatoes, then bake in the centre of a preheated oven at 180°C (gas mark 4) for 20 minutes.*
- *Serve immediately.*

*Carbohydrate content per serving: **7** grams*

**Stir-fried red cabbage with pine nuts**

For 2
3 tbsp extra-virgin olive oil
1 medium-sized brown onion, peeled and chopped
1 large garlic clove, peeled and chopped
½ red cabbage, finely sliced
2 tbsp white wine vinegar
1 tsp brown sugar
100 grams pine nuts
Freshly ground black pepper

- *Heat 2 tbsp of the extra-virgin olive oil in a medium frying pan and sauté the onion and garlic for 2–3 minutes.*
- *Add the red cabbage and stir-fry for 2–3 minutes.*
- *Stir in the white wine vinegar and sugar, and stir-fry for a further minute.*
- *Dry stir-fry the pine nuts for 1 minute.*
- *Stir the pine nuts into the cabbage, season to taste and serve immediately.*

*Carbohydrate content per serving: **9** grams*

**Tabbouleh**

For 2    40 grams bulgur (cracked) wheat
2 tbsp extra-virgin olive oil
3 tbsp freshly squeezed lemon juice
1 tbsp chopped fresh basil
1 tbsp chopped fresh mint
2 spring onions, finely chopped
Freshly ground black pepper

- *Soak the bulgur wheat for 25–30 minutes, then squeeze dry.*
- *Stir in the extra-virgin olive oil, lemon juice, basil, mint and chopped spring onions.*
- *Season to taste and serve.*

*Carbohydrate content per serving: **17** grams*

**Tzatziki**

For 2    4 tbsp Greek plain yoghurt
         1 tbsp chopped fresh mint leaves
         1 medium Lebanese cucumber, finely chopped
         Freshly ground black pepper
         Pinch of paprika

- *Mix together the yoghurt, mint and grated cucumber, and season to taste.*
- *Cool in the fridge for 2–4 hours, garnish with a pinch of paprika and serve immediately.*

*Carbohydrate content per serving:* **5** *grams*

## Sliced Brussels sprouts with ginger

For 2
2 tbsp extra-virgin olive oil
150 grams Brussels sprouts, finely sliced
3 slices of fresh ginger root, peeled and finely chopped
1 tsp sugar
1 tbsp light soy sauce
1 tbsp water
Freshly ground black pepper

- *Heat the extra-virgin olive oil in a wok.*
- *Add the Brussels sprouts and stir-fry for 1–2 minutes.*
- *Stir in the ginger, sugar, soy sauce and water, and stir-fry for about 3–4 minutes, then season to taste and serve immediately.*

*Carbohydrate content per serving: **6** grams*

**Green veggies with mustard sauce**

For 2   100 grams mangetout
100 grams broccoli florets
25 grams unsalted butter
25 grams flour
150 ml full-cream milk
1 tsp mustard powder
Freshly ground black pepper
1 tbsp chopped fresh parsley.

- *Place the mangetout and broccoli florets in a microwave-safe container, add 1 tbsp cold water, cover and cook on high for 2 minutes, then allow to stand for 1 minute.*

*Or*

- *Lightly steam the mangetout and broccoli for 4–5 minutes.*

*At the same time*

- *Melt the butter in a small saucepan, remove from the heat and stir in the flour.*
- *Return the pan to a gentle heat and gradually stir in the milk.*
- *Stir in the mustard powder.*

- *Serve the mustard sauce over the vegetables, season to taste and garnish with parsley.*

*Carbohydrate content per serving: **17** grams*

## Sautéed Halloumi with spinach

For 2     2 tbsp extra-virgin olive oil
80 grams Halloumi cheese, sliced
2 medium shallots, peeled and chopped
1 medium garlic clove, peeled and chopped
2 slices fresh ginger root, peeled and finely chopped
3 medium courgettes, sliced
100 grams fresh spinach leaves, washed
3 black olives, sliced
Freshly ground black pepper

- *Heat 1 tbsp of the extra-virgin olive oil in a medium frying pan and fry the Halloumi cheese for 3 minutes, turning once.*
- *Remove from the pan with a slotted spoon and set aside.*
- *Heat the remaining extra-virgin olive oil in the pan and stir-fry the shallots, garlic, ginger and courgettes for 2–3 minutes.*
- *Stir in the spinach leaves and stir-fry for a further minute.*
- *Serve immediately, topped with the Halloumi cheese and garnished with black olives, and season to taste.*

*Carbohydrate content per serving: 4 grams*

## Jerusalem artichokes with courgettes and leeks

For 2    1 tbsp extra-virgin olive oil
2 Jerusalem artichokes, chopped into 2–3 cm cubes
2 large courgettes, chopped into 2–3 cm chunks on
     the diagonal
1 medium leek, topped and tailed and chopped into
     2–3 cm rounds
1 garlic clove, peeled and finely chopped
25 grams button mushrooms, wiped and finely sliced
100 ml vegetable stock
1 tbsp chopped fresh coriander leaves
Freshly ground black pepper
1 tbsp double cream
1 tbsp chopped fresh chives, to garnish

- *Heat the extra-virgin olive oil in a medium frying pan and sauté the artichokes, leek, garlic and mushrooms for 2–3 minutes.*
- *Stir in the stock and coriander leaves, and simmer gently for 10 minutes (or until most of the stock has evaporated).*
- *Season to taste with freshly ground black pepper, stir in the cream and heat through gently for 1–2 minutes (do not boil!).*
- *Serve immediately, garnished with chopped fresh chives.*

*Carbohydrate content per serving: **16** grams*

### Sweet and sour shallots

For 2    2 tbsp extra-virgin olive oil
6 shallots, peeled and finely chopped
1 medium garlic clove, peeled and chopped
2 tsp caster sugar
3 tbsp freshly squeezed lemon juice
1 tsp Thai fish sauce
1 tbsp freshly chopped basil leaves
1 tbsp freshly chopped coriander leaves
2–3 drops Tabasco sauce (optional)

- *Heat the extra-virgin olive oil in a medium frying pan and sauté the shallots and garlic for 2–3 minutes.*
- *Stir in the sugar, lemon juice, fish sauce, basil, coriander and Tabasco sauce, gently simmer for 1–2 minutes, and serve.*

*Carbohydrate content per serving:* **14** *grams*

**Aubergines with sesame seeds**

For 2    1 tbsp sesame seeds
         4 tbsp extra-virgin olive oil
         1 large aubergine, chopped into 3–4 cm chunks
         1 tbsp soy sauce
         1 tbsp dry sherry
         1 tsp granulated sugar
         1 tsp sesame oil
         Freshly ground black pepper

- *Dry stir-fry the sesame seeds in a small saucepan for 1 minute, then remove from the pan and set aside.*
- *Heat the extra-virgin olive oil in a wok and stir-fry the aubergine for 3–4 minutes.*
- *Add the soy sauce, sherry and sugar, and stir-fry for about 2 minutes.*
- *Stir in the sesame oil, heat through for about a minute, then season to taste and serve immediately, garnished with toasted sesame seeds.*

*Carbohydrate content per serving:* **9** *grams*

### Steamed courgettes with garlic

For 2    150 grams courgettes, chopped on the diagonal into
2 cm cubes
25 grams unsalted butter
50 grams button mushrooms, wiped and halved
lengthways
1 medium garlic clove, peeled and finely chopped
Freshly ground black pepper

- *Lightly steam the courgettes for 5 minutes (or microwave on 'high' for 2–3 minutes).*
- *Melt the butter in a medium saucepan and sauté the mushrooms and garlic for 1–2 minutes.*
- *Serve the courgettes topped with mushrooms and garlic.*
- *Season to taste with freshly ground black pepper.*

*Carbohydrate content per serving: **3** grams*

**Spicy okra with pine nuts**

For 2   75 grams pine nuts

2 tsp sesame seeds

2 tbsp groundnut oil

1 medium garlic clove, peeled and finely chopped

2 slices of fresh ginger root, peeled and finely chopped

1 small red chilli, deseeded and finely chopped (optional)

100 grams okra, trimmed

1 tbsp fresh coriander leaves, to garnish

- *Dry stir-fry the pine nuts and sesame seeds in a medium frying pan for 1 minute, then set aside.*
- *Heat the groundnut oil in the pan and stir-fry the garlic, ginger, chilli and okra for 2–3 minutes.*
- *Stir in the pine nuts and sesame seeds, and stir-fry for a final 2 minutes.*
- *Serve immediately, garnished with fresh coriander leaves.*

*Carbohydrate content per serving: **7** grams*

### Chardonnay fennel with basil

For 2    1 large fennel bulb, stalk and outer leaves removed, then sliced
1 tbsp chopped fresh basil
75 ml vegetable stock
1 tbsp Chardonnay white wine
Freshly ground black pepper

- *Place the fennel, basil, stock and Chardonnay in a medium saucepan, bring to the boil and simmer gently for 20 minutes.*
- *Season to taste and serve immediately.*

*Carbohydrate content per serving: **8** grams*

**Green veggies and shallot purée**

For 2    150 grams Brussels sprouts, trimmed and quartered
           lengthways
         3 shallots, peeled and finely chopped
         1 small garlic clove, peeled and finely chopped
         2 slices fresh root ginger, peeled and finely chopped
         Freshly ground black pepper

- *Mix together the sprouts, shallots, garlic and ginger.*
- *Lightly steam the mixture for 7–8 minutes (or microwave on 'high' for 3–4 minutes).*
- *Blend together to make a purée.*
- *Season to taste and serve immediately.*

*Carbohydrate content per serving: **6** grams*

## Warm spinach with crème fraîche

For 2    25 grams unsalted butter
         150 grams fresh spinach leaves
         2 tbsp crème fraîche
         1 tbsp finely chopped fresh mint leaves
         Freshly ground black pepper

- *Melt the butter in a medium saucepan, stir in the spinach and cook for about a minute, stirring constantly, until the spinach just begins to wilt.*
- *Remove from the heat and stir in the crème fraîche and mint leaves.*
- *Season to taste and serve immediately.*

*Carbohydrate content per serving: **5** grams*

**Tangy wild rocket with orange**

For 2    25 grams unsalted butter
         150 grams wild rocket leaves
         3 tbsp freshly squeezed orange juice
         1 tbsp freshly squeezed lemon juice (optional)

- *Melt the butter in a medium saucepan, stir in the wild rocket leaves and cook for about a minute, stirring constantly, until the rocket just begins to wilt.*
- *Remove from the heat and stir in the orange and lemon juice.*
- *Serve immediately.*

*Carbohydrate content per serving: **6** grams*

**Traditional cauliflower cheese**

For 2    ½ medium cauliflower, washed and chopped into
            florets
         Pinch of rock salt
         Freshly ground black pepper
         15 grams Parmesan cheese, grated
         1 tbsp chopped fresh flat-leaf parsley

**Cheese sauce**

         25 grams butter
         25 grams wholemeal flour
         150 ml full-cream milk
         30 grams Cheddar cheese, grated

- *Place the cauliflower florets in a medium saucepan
  and add water until just covered.*
- *Add a pinch of rock salt, bring to the boil and simmer
  for 8–10 minutes.*

*At the same time*

- *Melt the butter in a medium saucepan, then remove
  from the heat and stir in the flour to form a smooth
  roux.*
- *Return to a gentle heat and gradually stir in the milk,
  stirring constantly.*
- *When the sauce begins to thicken, remove from the
  heat and stir in the Cheddar cheese.*
- *Return to the heat, stirring constantly, until the cheese
  has completely melted.*

- *Place the cauliflower florets on a grill-safe dish and
  pour over the cheese sauce.*
- *Season to taste with freshly ground black pepper,*

*sprinkle over the Parmesan cheese and grill under a hot grill (no closer than 8–10 cm from the grill) for 1–2 minutes until the Parmesan begins to brown.*

- *Sprinkle over the flat-leaf parsley and serve immediately.*

*Carbohydrate content per serving: 16 grams*

## Black olive tapenade

For 2   100 grams black stoneless olives
        1 tsp capers, rinsed
        1 anchovy fillet
        1 medium garlic clove, crushed
        Pinch of freshly ground black pepper
        2 tbsp extra-virgin olive oil

- *Blend together the olives, capers, anchovy, garlic and pepper.*
- *Gradually add the extra-virgin olive oil.*
- *Serve immediately.*

*Carbohydrate content per serving: **4** grams*

# Salads

### Sweet and sour courgettes

For 2    2 tsp sesame seeds
4 large courgettes, chopped on the diagonal
2 slices fresh ginger root, peeled and finely chopped
1 tsp sesame oil
2 tsp granulated sugar
1 tbsp white wine vinegar
Freshly ground black pepper

- *Dry stir-fry the sesame seeds in a small saucepan for 1 minute and set aside.*
- *Mix together the courgettes, ginger and sesame oil in a medium bowl.*
- *Dissolve the sugar in the wine vinegar, pour over the courgettes and marinate for 20–30 minutes, stirring frequently.*
- *Season to taste and garnish with toasted sesame seeds.*

*Carbohydrate content per serving:* **9 grams**

## Hummus with alfalfa

For 2     300 grams tinned chickpeas, drained
         1 small garlic clove, finely chopped
         1 tsp freshly squeezed lemon juice
         1 tbsp cold water
         1 tbsp chopped fresh basil
         3–4 drops Tabasco sauce
         30 grams alfalfa
         2 radishes, chopped
         1 large on-the-vine plum tomato, chopped
         1 Lebanese cucumber, sliced lengthways
         Pinch of paprika

- *Blend together the chickpeas, garlic, lemon juice, water, basil and Tabasco sauce.*
- *Toss the salad of alfalfa, radishes, tomato and cucumber.*
- *Spoon the hummus on a bed of alfalfa salad and sprinkle over a pinch of paprika.*

*Carbohydrate content per serving:* **30 grams**

**Baby leeks and macadamia nut salad**

For 2    6 baby leeks
50 grams macadamia nuts
75 grams wild rocket leaves
1 celery stick, chopped on the diagonal
25 grams freshly shaved Parmesan cheese
Freshly ground black pepper
Groundnut vinaigrette (page 222)

- *Lightly steam the baby leeks for 3–4 minutes (or microwave on 'high' for 2–3 minutes).*
- *Set aside to cool, then chop into 2–3 cm lengths on the diagonal.*
- *Mix together the leeks, macadamia nuts, wild rocket, celery and Parmesan in a large mixing bowl, and season to taste.*
- *Drizzle over a little Groundnut vinaigrette and serve immediately.*

*Carbohydrate content per serving: **6** grams*

## Roasted nut and cucumber radish salad

For 2    1 large cucumber, chopped into 2–3 cm cubes
3 radishes, finely sliced
1 fennel bulb, outer leaves removed, washed and
    finely sliced
1 tbsp dry roasted peanuts
Lemon vinaigrette (page 221)
Freshly ground black pepper

- *Mix together the cucumber, radishes, fennel and peanuts in a medium bowl.*
- *Drizzle over some Lemon vinaigrette, and season to taste.*

*Carbohydrate content per serving: **18** grams*

**Waldorf salad**

Classic salads are easily included in this diet because they consist of essentially healthy ingredients!

For 2
1 large chicken breast, skin removed
25 grams unsalted butter, cubed
1 medium apple, cored and finely sliced lengthways
2 celery sticks, finely sliced
25 grams walnuts
25 grams pine nuts
1 tbsp freshly squeezed lemon juice
4 tbsp mayonnaise
Freshly ground black pepper

- *Place the chicken breast in an oven-safe dish, dot with butter, cover with pierced aluminium foil and bake in the centre of a preheated oven at 180°C (gas mark 4) for 30–35 minutes.*
- *Set aside to cool, then chop into 2–3 cm cubes.*
- *Mix together the apple, celery, walnuts, pine nuts and cubed chicken in a medium bowl.*
- *Stir the lemon juice into the mayonnaise, then stir into the chicken mixture.*
- *Season to taste and serve immediately.*

*Carbohydrate content per serving: **9** grams*

## Grilled red mullet and avocado salad

For 2    4 medium red mullet, cleaned
Extra-virgin olive oil
1 medium Hass avocado, peeled, chopped and stone
    removed
8 cherry tomatoes, halved
1 tbsp chopped fresh flat-leaf parsley
50 grams wild rocket
Freshly ground black pepper
Lemon vinaigrette (page 221)

- *Brush the red mullet with extra-virgin olive oil, then place under a medium grill for 8 minutes, turning once.*
- *Toss the avocado, tomatoes, parsley and rocket, and season to taste with freshly ground black pepper.*
- *Drizzle over a little Lemon vinaigrette.*
- *Serve the mullet with the salad.*

*Carbohydrate content per serving: **6** grams*

**Fennel and herb salad**

For 2    1 bulb Florence fennel, washed and chopped
1 spring onion, chopped on the diagonal into 2–3 cm
   lengths
50 grams mangetout, topped and tailed
75 grams fresh watercress
1 tbsp chopped fresh basil
1 tbsp chopped fresh chives
Freshly ground black pepper
French vinaigrette

- *Toss the ingredients of the salad, season to taste with freshly ground black pepper and drizzle over a little vinaigrette.*
- *Serve immediately.*

*Carbohydrate content per serving: **8** grams*

**English cucumber with garden-fresh mint**

For 2     ½ English cucumber, very finely sliced
           2 tbsp natural yoghurt
           2 tbsp chopped fresh mint
           1 tbsp freshly squeezed lime juice
           Sprig of fresh mint

- *Place the cucumber in a colander and allow to drain for 20–30 minutes.*

*At the same time*

- *Mix together the yoghurt, mint and lime juice.*

- *Overlap the cucumber slices in a circle on the plate, top with the minted yoghurt and garnish with a sprig of fresh mint.*

*Carbohydrate content per serving: **6** grams*

**Fontina and olive salad**

For 2    75 grams Fontina cheese, finely sliced
         12 black olives, halved and stone removed
         ½ Cos lettuce, washed and leaves separated
         1 tbsp fresh basil leaves, washed
         Freshly ground black pepper

• *Toss the ingredients of the salad and season to taste.*

*Carbohydrate content per serving:* **4** *grams*

Other delicious low-GI/low-carb salads which have been described in our previous books include:

### The New High Protein Diet

- Avocado and mint
- Bocconcini and avocado
- Char-grilled pepper salad with herb mayonnaise
- Courgette and sour cream and basil
- Crispy green
- Cucumber and bean sprout
- Cucumber and chive
- Feta
- Guacamole
- Radish and basil
- Rocket and avocado
- Rocket and olive
- Tomato and avocado
- Tomato and coriander
- Tomato and Parmesan
- Tomato and mozzarella with mango dressing
- Tomato, ginger and orange
- Tomato salsa

### The New High Protein Diet Cookbook

- Avocado with crème fraîche
- Barbecue turkey
- Caper and olive
- Chicken and Bocconcini
- Chicken and cashew
- Chives and pepper
- Crab with herbs

- Fennel and tomato
- Green salad with herbs
- Lebanese salad
- Scallop and calamari
- Semi-dried tomatoes and herbs

**The New High Protein Healthy Fast Food Diet**

- Chicken and wild rocket
- Crispy herb
- Gazpacho
- Port salut, courgettes and chives
- Radicchio and cucumber
- Radish and mint
- Rocket and tofu

# Chapter 12 Delicious puddings

Desserts are usually the most difficult meals to incorporate into a low-carbohydrate diet because most of them consist primarily of refined carbohydrates and sugars! However, as we intend to incorporate *only* healthy ingredients in this healthy low-GI diet, we would naturally be replacing refined sugars with unrefined sugars (as in fruit) where possible. Obviously cakes, pastries, cheesecakes and sweets are denied by their very nature because they include large quantities of refined sugars and are therefore intrinsically unhealthy. This does not mean that you have to forgo these forever, merely during the weight-loss phase of the diet. You can reintroduce these delights into your diet – in moderation – after the weight-loss phase, but always remember that they are unhealthy and will definitely increase your insulin levels (and your weight) if they are consumed to excess.

So if we have to exclude all of the sweet, sugary desserts, does this inevitably mean that desserts are off the menu? Certainly not – it simply restricts us to healthy alternatives, such as summer berries with fresh cream, crème brûlée or fruit sorbet. And as the aim of this book is to include only the healthiest of ingredients, any restriction of excessive refined carbohydrates is certain to be healthy!

One possible solution is to use sugar substitutes in the recipes and this technique is employed by several authors. We have not taken this approach for several reasons: firstly, the aim of a *healthy* diet (which effectively means including all of the essential nutrients but reducing unhealthy, refined carbohydrates) should be to include only pure and unrefined ingredients, where possible; secondly, if you reduce all sweeteners (including low-carb sweeteners) you will naturally reduce your addiction to sweet flavours. By reducing your addiction to sweet flavours, you will naturally reduce your levels of insulin, which is essential for successful weight loss as insulin controls fat deposition.

### Baked egg custard

For 4      3 large free-range eggs
500 ml full-cream milk
1½ tbsp caster sugar
Freshly ground nutmeg

- *Beat together the eggs and milk.*
- *Strain the mixture through a sieve and stir in the caster sugar.*
- *Pour the mixture into a greased oven-safe dish.*
- *Sprinkle with freshly ground nutmeg.*
- *Place the dish in a roasting tin.*
- *Pour hot water into the roasting tin to about half the depth of the dish.*
- *Bake in the centre of a preheated oven at 160°C (gas mark 2) for 50–60 minutes, depending on the oven.*

*Carbohydrate content per serving: **13** grams*

## Lemon syllabub

For 2    75 ml dry white wine
1 tbsp freshly squeezed lemon juice
1 tsp finely grated lemon rind
1½ tbsp caster sugar
150 ml double cream
Fresh mint leaves, to garnish

- *Mix together the white wine, lemon juice, lemon rind and sugar in a medium bowl.*
- *Stir in the cream and spoon into wine glasses.*
- *Chill in the fridge for 2–3 hours and serve, garnished with fresh mint leaves.*

*Carbohydrate content per serving: **15** grams*

## Cointreau syllabub

For 2     1 tbsp Cointreau
1 tbsp caster sugar
4 tbsp freshly squeezed orange juice
100 ml fresh double cream
Pinch of ground nutmeg

- *Mix together the Cointreau, caster sugar and orange juice in a medium bowl and stir in the cream.*
- *Spoon the mixture into wine glasses and chill in the fridge for 2–4 hours.*
- *Sprinkle over a pinch of ground nutmeg and serve chilled.*

*Carbohydrate content per serving: **17** grams*

## Strawberries with blueberry purée

For 2    150 grams blueberries, washed
          2 tbsp water
          25 grams icing sugar
          100 ml double cream
          200 grams strawberries, washed and hulled

- *Place the blueberries, water and sugar in a medium saucepan and simmer for 4–5 minutes.*
- *Set aside to cool.*
- *Strain the blueberries to purée.*
- *Whip the double cream.*
- *Arrange the strawberries on dessert plates, top with whipped cream and drizzle the blueberry purée beside the strawberries.*
- *Serve immediately.*

*Carbohydrate content per serving: **30** grams*

## Crème brûlée

For 2    2 large free-range eggs
         150 ml double cream
         1 tbsp icing sugar
         ½ tsp vanilla essence
         1 tbsp caster sugar

- *Separate the yolks from the egg whites, and beat the yolks in a medium bowl.*
- *Pour the cream into a small saucepan and heat gently, but do not boil.*
- *Beat the cream into the beaten yolks.*
- *Stir in the icing sugar and vanilla essence.*
- *Pour the mixture into the saucepan and heat very gently (but do not allow to boil), stirring constantly until the mixture thickens.*
- *Pour into a 500 ml shallow, greased grill-safe dish and chill in the fridge for at least 4 hours (preferably overnight).*
- *Just before serving, sprinkle the caster sugar over the mixture, then grill under a medium grill, no closer than 8–10 cm from the grill, until the sugar caramelises.*
- *Remove from the heat and chill before serving.*

*Carbohydrate content per serving: **18** grams*

**Ricotta with soft berries**

For 2    100 grams blackberries, washed
        75 grams ricotta cheese, sliced
        2 tsp honey
        100 grams strawberries, washed, hulled and quartered
          lengthways
        Fresh mint leaves, to garnish (optional)

- *Purée the blackberries in a blender.*
- *Arrange the slices of ricotta cheese in the centre of the plates and drizzle over the honey.*
- *Drizzle the blackberry purée over the cheese.*
- *Top with strawberries and mint leaves.*

*Carbohydrate content per serving: **14** grams*

**Crêpes**

For 2    50 grams plain flour
         Pinch of salt
         1 large free-range egg, beaten
         150 ml full-cream milk
         1 tbsp melted butter

- *Sieve the flour and salt into a medium bowl.*
- *Add ½ of the beaten egg mixture, whisking constantly.*
- *Gradually blend in the milk, drawing the mixture to the centre of the bowl until you achieve an even consistency.*
- *Allow to stand for at least ½ hour before making the crêpes.*
- *Just before cooking, stir the melted butter into the mixture.*

Crêpes can be made by either the traditional method or by using a commercial crêpe-maker. Commercial crêpe-makers are not expensive and effectively allow crêpes to be included as an integral part of a quick low-carb diet.

**Traditional method**

- *Add a level teaspoon of butter to a small non-stick frying pan, melt the butter over a medium heat and evenly coat the pan.*
- *Add 2 tablespoons of the mixture to the pan, then tip the pan to evenly coat the base of the pan. Cook for about 20-30 seconds and remove with a pallete knife.*

**Crêpe-maker**

- *Pour the mixture into a wide shallow dish.*
- *Turn on the crêpe-maker. When hot, dip the crêpe-*

*maker horizontally onto the mixture to lightly coat and
allow the crêpe to cook. When the edge of the crêpe is
lightly browned, remove with a pallete spatula and
repeat the process.*

**Crêpes suzette**

For 2   6 crêpes
5 tbsp freshly squeezed orange juice
2 tbsp freshly squeezed lemon juice
2 tbsp Cointreau
1 tsp caster sugar
25 grams butter

- *Mix together the orange juice, lemon juice, Cointreau and sugar in a medium mixing bowl.*
- *Heat the butter in a medium frying pan and gently heat the sauce mixture.*
- *Lay a crêpe on the citrus mixture in the pan, allow the crêpe to absorb the mixture for about 30 seconds, then fold in half and remove from the pan.*
- *Add each of the other crêpes in a similar manner.*
- *Serve immediately.*

*Carbohydrate content per serving: **30** grams*

**Crêpes with apple and cinnamon**
To the recipe for Crêpes, add ½ tsp ground cinnamon and peeled and grated apple.

*Carbohydrate content per serving: **26** grams*

**Crêpes with lemon and cinnamon**
To the recipe for Crêpes, add ½ tsp ground cinnamon and drizzle 1 tbsp freshly squeezed lemon juice over each crêpe.

*Carbohydrate content per serving: **22** grams*

## Strawberries in raspberry cream

For 2    100 grams strawberries, washed and hulled, then
          halved lengthways
          Raspberry cream (page 214)

- *Stir the strawberries into the Raspberry cream and
  serve immediately.*

*Carbohydrate content per serving: **19** grams*

## Poached pears in Cabernet Sauvignon

For 2    250 ml Cabernet Sauvignon red wine
         25 grams caster sugar
         3 cloves
         2 large pears, washed and peeled
         Sprigs of fresh mint, to garnish

- *Pour the wine into a medium saucepan and stir in the sugar and cloves.*
- *Heat the wine, stirring constantly, until the sugar dissolves.*
- *Add the pears and simmer gently for 30 minutes, turning them occasionally.*
- *Remove the cloves, then serve the pears with the reduced red wine sauce, garnished with sprigs of fresh mint.*

*Carbohydrate content per serving: **30** grams*

## Soft berry brûlée

For 4    100 ml whipped cream
         100 ml natural yoghurt
         150 grams fresh raspberries, washed
         150 grams fresh blackberries (or blueberries), washed
         25 grams demerara sugar
         Fresh mint leaves, to garnish

* *Mix together the whipped cream and yoghurt.*
* *Place the berries in the base of a grill-safe shallow dish.*
* *Spread the cream and yoghurt mixture over the fruit and chill in the fridge for 1–2 hours.*
* *Sprinkle the sugar over the cream mixture and cook under a medium grill, no closer than 8–10 cm from the flame, until the sugar caramelises.*
* *Serve immediately, garnished with fresh mint leaves.*

*Carbohydrate content per serving: **16** grams*

**Dark chocolate mousse**

For 2   45 grams dark chocolate (minimum 70 per cent cocoa
content)
20 ml fresh full-cream milk
50 ml fresh double cream
4 fresh mint leaves, to garnish

- *Grate about 5 grams (very little) of the chocolate and set aside.*
- *Break up the chocolate into small pieces, place in a heat-safe bowl and lay the bowl over a pan of gently simmering hot water. Stir the chocolate from the edges of the bowl as it gradually melts.*
- *Heat the milk, then stir the milk into the chocolate.*
- *Set aside to cool.*
- *Whip the double cream until stiff, then fold the cream into the chocolate mixture.*
- *Transfer the chocolate mousse to ramekin dishes.*
- *Sprinkle a little grated chocolate over each dish, garnish with mint leaves and serve immediately.*

*Carbohydrate content per serving:* **10** *grams*

**Creamy vanilla (white) chocolate mousse**

For 2   As for Dark chocolate mousse (above), substituting
dark chocolate with vanilla chocolate.

*Carbohydrate content per serving:* **15** *grams*

## Crème caramel

For 2    75 ml water
2 ½ tbsp granulated sugar
2 large free-range eggs
½ tsp vanilla essence
250 ml full-cream milk
75 ml fresh single cream

- *Pour the water into a small saucepan and stir in 2 tbsp of the sugar.*
- *Heat over a low heat and stir constantly until the sugar has completely dissolved.*
- *Boil the mixture until the syrup turns a golden colour.*
- *Pour the syrup into a greased oven-safe dish.*
- *Tilt the dish to cover the base with the syrup.*
- *Whisk the eggs and stir in the vanilla essence and the remaining ½ tbsp sugar.*
- *Pour the milk into a small saucepan and heat gently until warm: do not boil.*
- *Stir in the whisked egg mixture.*
- *Sieve the mixture and pour into the caramelised dish.*
- *Place the oven-safe dish in a roasting tin, then pour sufficient hot water into the roasting tin to fill about half the depth of the dish.*
- *Cook in the centre of a preheated oven at 160°C (gas mark 2) for 50–60 minutes, depending on the oven.*
- *Remove from the oven and set aside to cool.*
- *Invert the dish onto a serving plate and serve with fresh cream.*

*Carbohydrate content per serving: **26** grams*

## Strawberry cream

For 2    1 tbsp caster sugar
       4 tbsp cold water
       200 grams fresh strawberries, washed and hulled
       200 ml whipped cream

- *Dissolve the sugar in the water in a small saucepan.*
- *Bring to the boil and simmer until reduced to about half.*
- *Add the strawberries (setting aside 4 strawberries for garnishing) and gently simmer for 5 minutes.*
- *Blend the mixture and set aside to cool.*
- *Fold the strawberry purée into the whipped cream.*
- *Spoon the mixture into dessert dishes.*
- *Quarter the remaining strawberries to garnish.*

*Carbohydrate content per serving: **17** grams*

## Raspberry cream

For 2    As for Strawberry cream (above), substituting
       raspberries for strawberries.

*Carbohydrate content per serving: **16** grams*

## Peach and blackberry surprise

For 2   150 grams ripe blackberries
2 ripe peaches, peeled, stone removed and halved
2 tsp freshly squeezed lime juice
100 ml single cream

- *Purée the blackberries, keeping 2 blackberries for garnish.*
- *Place the peach halves on two dessert plates and drizzle the lime juice over the peaches.*
- *Spoon the purée onto the plate next to the peaches.*
- *Pour some fresh cream over the peaches and top with a fresh blackberry.*
- *Serve immediately.*

*Carbohydrate content per serving:* **20** *grams*

**Lemon sorbet**

For 4   300 ml cold water
        75 grams granulated sugar
        6 tbsp freshly squeezed lemon juice
        1 tbsp grated lemon rind
        1 egg white
        15 grams caster sugar

- *Pour 100 ml of the water into a medium saucepan and stir in the granulated sugar.*
- *Heat the mixture over a low heat, stirring constantly until the sugar dissolves.*
- *Remove from the heat and strain the mixture.*
- *Stir in the remaining water, lemon juice and lemon rind.*
- *Pour the mixture into a suitable container and chill in the freezer for 20–30 minutes, then stir.*
- *Freeze the lemon mixture for a further 45–60 minutes.*
- *Beat the egg whites until stiff and whisk in the caster sugar.*
- *Whisk the lemon mixture and gradually fold in the egg white.*
- *Freeze for 30–40 minutes and whisk again.*
- *Freeze for 2–3 hours, then scoop the lemon sorbet into appropriate dessert dishes and serve immediately.*

*Carbohydrate content per serving:* **23** *grams*

### 'Zesty' fresh fruit salad

For 2  2 kiwi fruit, peeled and sliced
½ pink grapefruit, skin removed and chopped into
   segments
½ small mango, chopped
2 tbsp freshly squeezed lemon juice
1 tsp caster sugar
150 ml single cream
Sprigs of fresh mint, to garnish

- *Mix together the kiwi fruit, grapefruit segments, mango, lemon juice and sugar in a medium bowl.*
- *Cool in the fridge for 30–60 minutes.*
- *Serve with single cream, garnished with a sprig of mint.*

*Carbohydrate content per serving: **27** grams*

**Strawberries with Cointreau**

For 2     200 grams fresh strawberries, washed and hulled
          3 tbsp Cointreau
          6 tbsp freshly squeezed orange juice
          200 ml double cream
          Fresh mint leaves, to garnish

- *Mix together the strawberries, Cointreau and orange juice, cover and chill in the fridge for 2 hours.*
- *Transfer the mixture to dessert dishes and top with cream.*
- *Garnish with fresh mint leaves and serve immediately.*

*Carbohydrate content per serving: **18** grams*

**Red fruit fool**

For 2    150 grams mixed fruit: raspberries, redcurrants and
         rhubarb (chopped)
         4 tbsp water
         25 grams caster sugar
         1 tbsp freshly squeezed lemon juice
         150 ml fresh double cream
         4 fresh mint leaves, to garnish

* *Place the mixed fruit, water, sugar and lemon juice in
  a medium saucepan, bring to the boil, then lower the
  heat and simmer gently until the fruit softens.*
* *Blend until smooth and set aside to cool.*
* *Whisk the cream until firm and fold into the purée.*
* *Transfer to a medium bowl and chill before serving,
  garnished with fresh mint leaves.*

*Carbohydrate content per serving: **18** grams*

**Custard fruit fool**

For 2    As for Red fruit fool (above), substituting cream with
         custard.

*Carbohydrate content per serving: **28** grams*

**Yoghurt fruit fool**

For 2    As for Red fruit fool (above), substituting cream with
         Greek yoghurt.

*Carbohydrate content per serving: **23** grams*

**Zabaglione**

For 2    4 medium free-range egg yolks
         4 tsp caster sugar
         2 tbsp Marsala wine (or medium sherry)

- *Place the egg yolks and caster sugar in a medium heat-safe mixing bowl and whisk together until smooth.*
- *Gradually add the Marsala or sherry, whisking constantly.*
- *Add sufficient water to a large saucepan to a depth of 3–4 cm, then heat until the water is gently simmering.*
- *Place the heat-safe mixing bowl in the saucepan of gently simmering water and continue to whisk until the mixture thickens, but be very careful not to overheat.*
- *When the mixture begins to thicken, pour into wine glasses and serve immediately.*

*Carbohydrate content per serving: **12** grams*

# Chapter 13 Dressings and sauces

Dressings and sauces are an essential ingredient in the enjoyment of food. Salads are transformed by a drizzle of tangy dressing or a dollop of delicious mayonnaise. Can you imagine lasagne without white sauce, or roast turkey without gravy? Sauces, salsas, chutneys and pestos are an integral feature of the enjoyment of food. More importantly, the basic ingredients of these accompaniments are very healthy foods. Extra-virgin olive oil in dressings and mayonnaise, avocados and chilli in guacamole, basil and pine nuts in pesto . . . the list is only as finite as the next sauce you prepare. In this and previous books we have described 46 different accompaniments, but you can probably add many more from your own repertoire.

## Lemon vinaigrette

For 4    4 tbsp extra-virgin olive oil
1 tbsp white wine vinegar
2 tbsp freshly squeezed lemon juice
Freshly ground black pepper

• *Mix together the ingredients in a screw-top jar.*

*Carbohydrate content per serving: 2 grams*

## Balsamic vinaigrette

For 2    4 tbsp extra-virgin olive oil
1 tbsp balsamic vinegar
1 tbsp chopped fresh flat-leaf parsley
Freshly ground black pepper

- *Mix together the ingredients in a screw-top jar.*

*Carbohydrate content per serving: 2 grams*

## Groundnut vinaigrette

For 2    4 tbsp groundnut oil
1 tbsp white wine vinegar
½ clove garlic, peeled and finely chopped
Freshly ground black pepper

- *Mix together the ingredients in a screw-top jar.*

*Carbohydrate content per serving: 1 gram*

## Mustard vinaigrette

For 4    4 tbsp extra-virgin olive oil
1 tbsp white wine vinegar
1 tbsp wholegrain mustard
1 small garlic clove, peeled and finely chopped

- *Mix together the ingredients in a screw-top jar.*

*Carbohydrate content per serving: 1 gram*

**Mustard and chive mayonnaise**

For 4
1 large free-range egg yolk, whisked
1½ tbsp Dijon mustard
½ tbsp granulated sugar
6 tbsp extra-virgin olive oil
1 tbsp white wine vinegar
1 tbsp finely chopped fresh chives
Freshly ground black pepper

- *Whisk together the egg yolk, mustard and sugar.*
- *Add the extra-virgin olive oil, drop by drop, whisking constantly.*
- *Stir in the white wine vinegar and chopped chives, and season to taste.*

*Carbohydrate content per serving:* **2** *grams*

## Horseradish and crème fraîche

For 4    150 ml crème fraîche
3 tbsp freshly squeezed lemon juice
1 tbsp horseradish, grated

- *Mix together the ingredients in a small bowl, cover and set aside to cool in the fridge for 1–2 hours before use.*

*Carbohydrate content per serving: **6** grams*

**Satay sauce**

For 4   1 tbsp groundnut oil
2 shallots, peeled and finely chopped
1 medium garlic clove, peeled and chopped
½ tsp ground cumin
½ tsp ground coriander
¼ tsp chilli powder (optional)
50 ml coconut milk
50 ml natural yoghurt
75 grams roasted (unsalted) peanuts

- *Heat the groundnut oil in a small saucepan and sauté the shallots and garlic for 2–3 minutes.*
- *Transfer to a blender, add the cumin, coriander, chilli, coconut milk, yoghurt and peanuts, and blend for 15–20 seconds.*

*Carbohydrate content per serving: **10** grams*

**Red pepper coulis**

For 2    2 large red peppers, deseeded and quartered
lengthways
2 tbsp extra-virgin olive oil
2 shallots, peeled and finely chopped
1 medium garlic clove, peeled and finely chopped
1 tbsp freshly squeezed orange juice
150 ml crème fraîche
Freshly ground black pepper

- *Place the peppers (skin uppermost) in a single layer on an oven tray, brush with 1 tbsp of the extra-virgin olive oil and cook in the centre of a preheated oven at 180°C (gas mark 4) for 20 minutes.*
- *Allow to cool, then peel the peppers.*

*At the same time*
- *Heat the remaining 1 tbsp extra-virgin olive oil in a small saucepan and sauté the shallots and garlic for 2–3 minutes.*
- *Set aside to cool.*

- *Add both the peppers and the shallot mixture to a blender and purée.*
- *Stir in the orange juice and crème fraîche, and season to taste.*

*Carbohydrate content per serving: **14** grams*

## Ginger salsa

For 4
1 tbsp extra-virgin olive oil
1 tsp sesame oil
3 slices fresh root ginger, peeled and grated
1 small red chilli, deseeded and finely chopped
1 tbsp freshly chopped basil leaves
1 tbsp freshly chopped coriander leaves
1 tbsp freshly squeezed lemon juice
Freshly ground black pepper

- *Mix together the ingredients of the salsa in a medium bowl and cool in the fridge for 2–3 hours before serving.*

*Carbohydrate content per serving: **2** grams*

**Coriander chutney**

For 4    2 tbsp fresh coriander leaves, washed
2 shallots, peeled and chopped
1 red chilli, deseeded and chopped
1 tsp garam masala
1 tbsp freshly squeezed lemon juice
2 tbsp crème fraîche
2 tbsp water

- *Blend all the ingredients until smooth.*
- *Chill for 1–2 hours before serving.*

*Carbohydrate content per serving: 3 grams*

**Cheese and bean dip**

Broad beans are particularly well suited to a low-carbohydrate diet as they contain only 6 grams of carbohydrate per 100 grams, but have all of the essential nutrients and amino acids present in pulses.

For 2
150 grams fresh  broad beans
75 grams Philadelphia cheese
1 small garlic clove, crushed
1 tbsp freshly squeezed lemon juice
1 tbsp chopped fresh basil leaves
Freshly ground black pepper
1 medium raw carrot, peeled and chopped into matchsticks
2 celery sticks

- *Lightly steam the broad beans for 5–6 minutes (or microwave on 'high' for 2–3 minutes).*
- *Peel the broad beans.*
- *Blend the beans with the cheese, garlic, lemon juice and basil, and season to taste.*
- *Serve immediately with carrot and celery.*

*Carbohydrate content per serving: **5 grams***

Once again, these dressings and sauces are complementary to the many others previously described in:

### The New High Protein Diet Cookbook

**Dressings**

French vinaigrette
Balsamic vinaigrette
Mint and chives vinaigrette
Honey and orange vinaigrette
Lemon and coriander vinaigrette
Oriental vinaigrette
Passata vinaigrette

**Mayonnaise**

Mayonnaise
Aioli
Herb mayonnaise
Hot mayonnaise
Chilli mayonnaise
Creamy curry mayonnaise

**Sauces**

Basic white sauce
Béchamel sauce
Basil and chive sauce
Leek and lemon butter sauce

Chilli and ginger sauce
Chilli tomato sauce
Basil pesto sauce
Basil and macadamia pesto sauce
Coriander pesto sauce
Red pesto sauce
Satay sauce
Capsicum and basil sauce
Coriander and basil sauce
Barbecue marinade
Mango and ginger chutney
Caper and basil marinade
Cucumber raita
Coriander and lemon butter
Horseradish sauce
Watercress and mint sauce
Gravy
Mint sauce
Apple sauce

# Chapter 14 Four-week meal plan

The most important feature of this diet is that it is healthy and flexible! This means that you have the option of choosing the foods that *you* enjoy and incorporating those foods into a healthy diet. So when we suggest a four-week menu for a healthy diet, this is obviously only a suggestion: we *know* that no one will follow this plan exactly because it is deliberately designed to incorporate a wide range of different tastes in food. It is designed to allow each dieter to *choose* those features which they most enjoy and to include those in their diet. We are all unique individuals with different tastes and lifestyles. The only way to ensure a diet perfectly tailored to the individual is to discuss preferences in a clinical setting and prepare a menu plan on that basis – which is exactly how we design healthy diets for our patients in our clinics. No book can attempt to provide a perfect menu for every different taste: however, we can provide a guideline to allow you to choose the types of foods which *you* enjoy and which can be included in your diet.

We have not described a different menu for breakfast, lunch and dinner for every day of the four-week period because this is not normal. As creatures of habit, we all have different lifestyles and we tend to have repetition in our meal habits. For example, many individuals will always have a cooked breakfast whilst many others never have a cooked breakfast. The items in this four-week plan are designed as a guide only. Provided you vary your diet and keep the daily carb limit within 50 grams, you will lose weight and increase your healthy parameters successfully.

All of the following recipes are described in the New High Protein Diet series: *The New High Protein Diet*, *The New High Protein Diet Cookbook*, *The New High Protein Healthy Fast Food Diet* and, of course, *The Healthy Low GI Low Carb Diet*. The wide variety of healthy and delicious foods which are included in this successful weight-loss diet are instantly apparent from the diversity of the potential menus.

Whether you prefer eggs, porridge, fresh fruit, kippers, cheese, fruit juices, smoothies, crêpes or continental-style breakfast, the choice is yours. Vary or repeat the various options in the following suggested menu plans according to your individual taste.

For lunch and dinner, whether self-prepared or as part of a hectic, busy lifestyle, the potential variations are almost infinite! We have deliberately included a selection from the many dishes which include pasta, rice, fish, shellfish, salads and vegetarian dishes described in the series to demonstrate how this healthy diet can be adapted to literally every lifestyle. Naturally, we do not expect everyone to have similar tastes in all of these various options: some may be overtly vegetarian whilst others may specifically dislike vegetarian meals. Some may dislike (or be allergic to) shellfish and others may prefer pasta on a semi-regular basis. This diet caters for all, but you must remember to *vary* your diet to obtain all of the essential nutrients from the different categories of foods, all of which have their individual strengths and weaknesses in regard to nutritional content. It is important to realise that no food is nutritionally perfect.

On some of the dinner menus we have included dessert. As you will appreciate, desserts may be easily incorporated into the programme, provided you count the carbs. By definition, desserts will always contain more carbs than many other foods but if you combine them in a daily menu with other low-carb meals (i.e. *not* with pasta and rice dishes, obviously) it is relatively simple to include delicious and healthy desserts on a regular basis.

All of the following recipes are available either in this book or in our previous books in the series.

## Week 1

**Breakfast:** Citrus smoothie (page 58)
1 large free-range boiled egg

**Lunch:** Angel hair pasta with Italian sauce (page 87)

**Dinner:** Fresh rainbow trout with caper butter (page 120)

*Carbohydrate total per day: **41** grams*

· · · · · · · · · · · · · · · · · · · · · · · · · · · · · · · · · · · · · · · · · · · · · · · · · · · · · · · · · · ·

**Breakfast:** Porridge (page 59)

**Lunch:** Avocado with Bocconcini salad lunchbox

**Dinner:** Griddled duck with lentil purée (pages 104–5)

*Carbohydrate total per day: **43** grams*

· · · · · · · · · · · · · · · · · · · · · · · · · · · · · · · · · · · · · · · · · · · · · · · · · · · · · · · · · · ·

**Breakfast:** Fresh fruit with natural yoghurt (page 59)

**Lunch:** Egg mayonnaise with fresh basil and chives

**Dinner:** Coconut okra curry (page 103)
Lemon syllabub (page 201)

*Carbohydrate total per day: **44** grams*

· · · · · · · · · · · · · · · · · · · · · · · · · · · · · · · · · · · · · · · · · · · · · · · · · · · · · · · · · · ·

**Breakfast:**   Sun-dried tomatoes and herb bagel

**Lunch:**   Scallop and calamari salad

**Dinner:**   Skate with pepper sauce
Peach and blackberry surprise (page 215)

*Carbohydrate total per day: **47** grams*

...........................................................

**Breakfast:**   Mint and cucumber smoothie (page 56)
Kippers with tomatoes (page 64)

**Lunch:**   Bocconcini and avocado salad

**Dinner:**   Chow mein (pages 111–12)

*Carbohydrate total per day: **49** grams*

...........................................................

**Breakfast:**   Char-grilled mushrooms with scrambled eggs
(page 63)

**Lunch:**   Mozzarella chicken

**Dinner:**   Milanese risotto (page 121)

*Carbohydrate total per day: **37** grams*

...........................................................

**Breakfast:**   Continental breakfast

**Lunch:**   Waldorf salad (page 191)

**Dinner:**   Balti chicken with tzatziki
Crème brûlée (page 204)

*Carbohydrate total per day: **43** grams*

## Week 2

**Breakfast:**   Avocado on toast

**Lunch:**   Chicken tikka salad lunchbox

**Dinner:**   Spicy prawns with rocket
Crêpes suzette (page 208)

*Carbohydrate total per day:* **50** *grams*

........................................................

**Breakfast:**   Tomatoes and poached eggs

**Lunch:**   Penne rigate with mixed veggies (page 90)

**Dinner:**   Barbary duck with teriyaki sauce (pages 107–8)
Soft berry brûlée (page 211)

*Carbohydrate total per day:* **46** *grams*

........................................................

**Breakfast:**   Baked haddock with grilled Swiss cheese

**Lunch:**   Greek salad

**Dinner:**   Button mushroom and basil risotto (page 140)
Peach and blackberry surprise (page 215)

*Carbohydrate total per day:* **49** *grams*

**Breakfast:**   Berry surprise smoothie (page 56)
Continental breakfast

**Lunch:**   Sesame tiger prawns with Chinese leaves
(page 91)

**Dinner:**   Char-grilled tofu kebabs with satay sauce
(page 155)

*Carbohydrate total per day: **47** grams*

...........................................................

**Breakfast:**   Omelette with basil and spring onion

**Lunch:**   Chicken drumsticks

**Dinner:**   Pan-fried cod with herb butter (page 102)
Crème caramel (page 213)

*Carbohydrate total per day: **32** grams*

...........................................................

**Breakfast:**   Porridge (page 59)

**Lunch:**   Tuna mayonnaise salad lunchbox

**Dinner:**   Barbecued turkey keftas with cucumber raita
Strawberries with Cointreau (page 218)

*Carbohydrate total per day: **46** grams*

**Breakfast:**   Sardines with herbs

**Lunch:**   Carrot and coriander soup

**Dinner:**   Ratatouille (page 158)
Zabaglione (page 220)

*Carbohydrate total per day: **40** grams*

## Week 3

**Breakfast:**   Fresh fruit with natural yoghurt (page 59)

**Lunch:**   Avocado with Bocconcini salad lunchbox

**Dinner:**   Poached salmon with lemon butter sauce
Dark chocolate mousse (page 212)

*Carbohydrate total per day: **43** grams*

..................................................................

**Breakfast:**   Continental breakfast

**Lunch:**   Hot fettuccine with basil and chicken (pages
117–8)

**Dinner:**   Rocket and tofu salad

*Carbohydrate total per day: **36** grams*

..................................................................

**Breakfast:**   Poached eggs with tomato

**Lunch:**   Lasagne (pages 129–30)

**Dinner:**   Sliced turkey with orange and basil (page 110)
Red fruit fool (page 219)

*Carbohydrate total per day: **48** grams*

**Breakfast:**    Blueberry milkshake
                  Kipper

**Lunch:**        Avocado soup

**Dinner:**       Ricotta soufflé (page 160)

*Carbohydrate total per day: 36 grams*

..........................................................

**Breakfast:**    Porridge (page 59)

**Lunch:**        Trout with lemon and pine nuts

**Dinner:**       Warm spinach curry (page 114)

*Carbohydrate total per day: 37 grams*

..........................................................

**Breakfast:**    Continental breakfast

**Lunch:**        Open sandwich with chicken and Swiss cheese

**Dinner:**       Smoked haddock kedgeree (page 145)

*Carbohydrate total per day: 41 grams*

**Breakfast:** Fresh fruit with natural yoghurt (page 59)

**Lunch:** Mascarpone and spinach soup (page 78)

**Dinner:** Lemon chicken with cashew nuts
Creamy vanilla chocolate mousse (page 212)

*Carbohydrate total per day:* **40** *grams*

**Week 4**

**Breakfast:** Scrambled eggs and mushrooms

**Lunch:** Waldorf salad (page 191)

**Dinner:** Tagliatelli Carbonara (page 127)
Peach and blackberry surprise (page 215)

*Carbohydrate total per day: **48** grams*

...........................................................

**Breakfast:** Porridge (page 59)

**Lunch:** Spicy crab with mango (page 142)

**Dinner:** Caponata

*Carbohydrate total per day: **43** grams*

...........................................................

**Breakfast:** Haddock and Parmesan crêpe

**Lunch:** Fennel and herb salad

**Dinner:** Chicken korma

*Carbohydrate total per day: **39** grams*

**Breakfast:**   Continental breakfast

**Lunch:**   Hot and spicy tomato soup (page 77)

**Dinner:**   Nasi Goreng (page 163)

*Carbohydrate total per day: **44** grams*

. . . . . . . . . . . . . . . . . . . . . . . . . . . . . . . . . . . . . . . . . . . . . . . . . . . .

**Breakfast:**   Fresh fruit with natural yoghurt (page 59)

**Lunch:**   Barbecue chicken with salad

**Dinner:**   Swordfish steaks with lemon and garlic

*Carbohydrate total per day: **31** grams*

. . . . . . . . . . . . . . . . . . . . . . . . . . . . . . . . . . . . . . . . . . . . . . . . . . . .

**Breakfast:**   Toasted cheese with mixed herbs

**Lunch:**   Mulligatawny soup

**Dinner:**   Tomato and coriander pappardelle

*Carbohydrate total per day: **49** grams*

**Breakfast:** Omelette

**Lunch:** Scallops with lime and ginger

**Dinner:** Char-grilled aubergines with peppers
'Zesty' fresh fruit salad (page 217)

*Carbohydrate total per day: **47** grams*

# Index